THE
PERFECT BALANCE
DIET

Barbara —
With love &
gratitude !

Jissa
Coffey

THE
PERFECT BALANCE
DIET

4 Weeks to a Lighter Body, Mind, Spirit & Space

By Lissa Coffey

Foreword by Valencia Porter, MD, MPH

The Perfect Balance Diet: 4 Weeks to a Lighter Body, Mind, Spirit & Space
Copyright © 2013 Lissa Coffey
Foreword ©2013 Valencia Porter
Published by
Bamboo Entertainment, Inc.
4607 Lakeview Canyon Road Suite 181
Westlake Village, CA 91361

ISBN-13: 978-0615847924

To Bhuvaneswari
And the Goddess within
Each One of us.

Praise for The Perfect Balance Diet

"Lissa Coffey has created a treasure of a handbook with countless practical suggestions based on the teachings of Ayurveda, showing us how we can eat, live, sleep, and interact with other people to find and maintain a balanced lifestyle. When we are naturally in balance, as Lissa suggests, we feel good, look good, and do good."

- **Lothar Schäfer, author,** *Infinite Potential: What Quantum Physics Reveals About How We Should Live*

"Our busy lives can take a toll on our health, and our weight. Lissa Coffey shows us how to get back into balance with timeless principles that we can use every single day. Brilliant!"

- **Mallika Chopra,** Founder of Intent.com

"Lissa Coffey's book puts health back into the word "diet". Using the ancient teachings of Ayurveda, she shows you how to make positive changes in both your diet and your life to move in the direction of greater health. Lissa's book is a welcome resource for every health and wellness library."

- **Sarah Maria, author,** *Love Your Body, Love Your Life.*

"Lissa Coffey walks her talk, and now has written a beautiful and clear book to teach us the most advanced and ancient ideas about achieving the perfect balance that results in the kind of health that helps us look, feel and be our very blessed best! She is an amazing woman and I am thrilled to recommend her book!"

- **Candace Pert, PhD, author,** *Molecules of Emotion: The Science Behind Mind-Body Medicine*

CONTENTS

Foreword	by Valencia Porter, MD, MPH	8
Intro		9
Chapter 1	The Balancing Act	14
Chapter 2	Food	22
Chapter 3	Sleep and Relationships	43
Chapter 4	House, Home, Haven	53
Chapter 5	Beauty Inside and Out	71
Chapter 6	Unplugged	87
Chapter 7	Weight Management	104
Chapter 8	The 28-Day Program	122
Chapter 9	Recipes for an Enlightened Lifestyle	167
Afterword		229
About the Author		231
Acknowledgements		233
References and Recommended Reading		234
Resources		236

FOREWORD

In this wonderful and informative book, The Perfect Balance Diet: 4 Weeks to a Lighter Body, Mind, Spirit & Space, written by Chopra Certified Instructor and relationship expert Lissa Coffey, readers are inspired and encouraged to bring balance into their lives and return to their true essence of health and wholeness. With compassion and humor, Lissa provides readers with a life guide for mind, body and spirit, far beyond just a diet book. The practical tools offered in this book enable us to know our inherent nature, so that we can personalize the recommendations to be our best selves. This is a book about listening to our inner wisdom and celebrating our individuality, rather than depriving ourselves of the satisfaction of life. It incorporates the ancient wisdom of Ayurvedic lifestyle techniques to optimize our health, paying particular attention to not only what we eat, but also how we eat and how to enhance our digestive capacities.

Having guided thousands of patients in these techniques at the Chopra Center for Wellbeing in Carlsbad, California, I have personally seen the benefit of the approaches outlined in this book. It is my belief that understanding one's true nature and utilizing the tools for balance described in this book will allow the reader to gain improved health and vitality in mind, body, and spirit. Many of my patients have found that this type of lifestyle approach has allowed them to have a more comfortable relationship with their body and with food and to achieve a naturally balanced weight. Others have finally gotten restful sleep or solved their digestive problems without having to rely on prescription medications. Whole person balance also means being in mutually nourishing relationships and having the ability to manifest our intentions and desires. If you are excited to embrace all that nature has bestowed upon you, I encourage you to allow the wisdom in these pages to guide you in this journey.

Valencia Porter, MD, MPH
Director of Integrative Medicine
The Chopra Center for Wellbeing
Carlsbad, California

INTRODUCTION

Imagine you're outside, by a beautiful lake, enjoying the perfection of your surroundings. You feel comfortable, relaxed, as if you are an important part of it all. You are so in tune that it is as if you can hear nature speaking to you.

You see a swan glide past, and the swan is thinking to itself: "How wonderful it is to be a swan. I can take my time; life is serene. I am graceful and lovely. All is right with the world."

And then you notice an eagle flying high overhead, and the eagle is thinking: "Ah, what a joy it is to be an eagle. I am strong, and free. This is the life!"

A hummingbird flits past, and you can hear the hummingbird is thinking: "I'm having so much fun on this glorious day. There's so much to see and do. I'm so glad I'm a hummingbird and can move easily to all the things I love."

Everything in nature has a purpose. We're all connected. Sitting amongst the trees and looking at the clear blue sky you know that you are an important part of this connection. You breathe deeply and feel an overwhelming sense of gratitude and peace. Now, imagine you're in that same place, same time. When you hear nature speaking to you things are a bit different.

You see a swan glide past, and the swan thinks to itself: "Oh, my. Why am I stuck being a swan? I would so much rather be like that little hummingbird. I want to flit around like that! I feel so dumpy just floating here on this silly lake."

Then the eagle flies overhead, and you read its thoughts: "Wow. Look at that swan down there. He's got the good life. Why can't I just hang out on the lake? Instead I'm up here working so hard. This isn't fair. I'd rather be a swan."

Then the hummingbird flits by and thinks: "Really? That eagle is so lucky. She's way up there with a great vantage point. She can go so far without even flapping her wings. I'm down here pumping away a million beats a minute! Man, I want to be an eagle."

Somehow, this second scenario just doesn't make sense, does it? Because this is not how nature operates! And yet, this is exactly what we do as human beings all the time. We fight our own nature. We compare ourselves to one another. We think we need to always be thinner, more beautiful, more successful, more something, anything! When the truth is that we are inherently perfect. If we are carrying around excess weight, or stress, or feeling bad about ourselves it is because we are out of balance, our lives are out of balance in one way or another. We can find that perfect state of balance, and regain our strength and confidence and energy to be the best that we can be.

The most important thing we can do for ourselves, to be our healthiest and happiest, body, mind, and spirit, is to know who we are. Some of us are swans, some of us are eagles, and some of us are hummingbirds. Each being is valid, each being has value, and each being brings his or her unique gifts to the world. When we know ourselves, and our own nature, we allow the best of ourselves to shine through. Nature operates through us. So why are we fighting it?

The goal of the Perfect Balance Diet is to help you be the best YOU that you can be. Honestly, "skinny" isn't for everyone! It would be like trying to get that swan to fly like a hummingbird. It would be totally against that swan's nature and only cause frustration to even attempt such a thing. The idea is to feel good – to be healthy, beautiful, have tons of energy, and be happy and comfortable in our own skin. When we are at this point in our lives, then we are naturally at our ideal weight.

A big part of achieving perfect balance is knowing that "perfect" is not some specific number or size or any one particular thing. We're not striving to be some image that we cut out and put on the refrigerator. The Perfect Balance Diet is about understanding that we are each perfect in our imperfections, in our unique qualities. Our flaws, quirks, and idiosyncrasies help to make us the beautifully imperfect beings that we are. We are perfect in our imperfections! There is an ancient art from Japan called "kintsukuroi." Kintsukuroi is the art of repairing broken or cracked pottery with gold or silver lacquer and understanding that the piece is more beautiful for having been broken. Yes, there are changes we want to make to our lives, and we know that these changes aren't to "fix" ourselves, they are to let our natural beauty shine through in every way.

More than a diet, The Perfect Balance Diet is a lifestyle shift. It's not a one-size-fits all solution, but rather a very personalized program that keeps us in balance. We don't need to create a "new you" – we need to bring you into balance to be your best you – the you that you already are but may not even know it!

There are a lot of things that take us away from our state of balance. We are overstressed and overworked. We overeat, and are overweight. We over exert ourselves, and overspend so that we end up tired, hungry, in debt and living in a mess. Look at all the extra "stuff" we carry around with us. We need to lighten up! We need to shed the stress, the pounds, the debt, and the distractions and focus on what is good for us, what serves us. Food is a huge part of all this. We use food to soothe our emotions, to fill up our tummies when we feel a lack in some part of our lives. We fall into habits, with food and otherwise, that we think are easy, and they become mindless and robotic so that we don't see any other possibilities or potential for ourselves.

Maybe you've tried some of the many diets that are out there, had some success, only to gain back all the weight. Most of these diets put excess strain on us. We have to count calories, get on the scale, monitor portions, and restrict ourselves with unrealistic limits. The Perfect Balance Diet is not about any of that! This is not about depriving yourself. This is not about losing weight, but rather about gaining balance. It is about celebrating yourself! It is about honoring you, and loving yourself. It's about listening to your body, following your instincts, and living in harmony with nature. The Perfect Balance Diet is about taking care of yourself so that you can express the true you, looking good, feeling great, functioning optimally and absolutely loving life!

In The Perfect Balance Diet you will learn about Ayurveda, the 5,000 year old Science of Life. You will learn how to identify your unique dosha, or mind/body type, so that you can customize your lifestyle so that you can be your very best. I'll get you started on a 28-day program that you can use as a template for living for the rest of your life.

The ancient Indian texts explain that there is much more to us than our physical bodies. There are four areas of our being that make up who we are, and how we live. No "diet" is complete if we are looking just at our physical body. We need to take a holistic approach and address all four areas of life: body, mind, spirit, and space. We have to look at what we are eating, what foods we are taking in, what nourishment we are giving our physical bodies. We also need to look at what we are taking in mentally, intellectually, what we are thinking, what we are learning, what images we look at, how we spend our time. We need to look at our relationships, and our activities. We need to understand how the choices we make affect our feelings and emotions. And we also need to look at our space, our environment, which is also our extended body. The energy in this space affects the other aspects of our lives in profound ways. What do we surround ourselves with? How do we care for our space? How is this indicative of how we care for ourselves in other ways?

The Perfect Balance Diet brings all of this together into a routine that you can integrate into your life and use every single day. You'll learn about how to express your personal style, and to create a healthy and happy environmental space – at home, in your office, anywhere you go. I'll show you how to give your kitchen a make-over, and give you recipes for meals that feed your body and soul.

We've got a four-week plan – one week for each of the four areas of life. Just 28 days where when we stick to a balanced routine we start getting used to how feeling good really feels. These four weeks will help to get some good habits going, so that we are eating, thinking, behaving and expressing in a more mindful, healthy, nurturing way. Throughout this book and as days go on you'll see how the scales are tipping back into balance and that you are becoming, or getting back to being, that person you were always meant to be, the real you. We feel lighter, not just in terms of weight but in terms of attitude. The world is just a little brighter, we feel a little less burdened, we feel a little freer.

After you've read the book, and incorporated the plan into your lifestyle, you may want to join our club, where you'll get menus, recipes, shopping lists, meditations, videos, and lots more. It's a great way to make Perfect Balance a part of your life every day. Check out our website for all the information: www.PerfectBalanceDiet.com "Dharma" is a Sanskrit word meaning "purpose." The Perfect Balance Diet is meant to help you fulfill your purpose, to express your unique talents, to contribute to the world, and to feel good about yourself body, mind, spirit and space. There's no better time to start than right now, no better place than right here. Let's go!

CHAPTER 1

THE BALANCING ACT

The best and safest thing is to keep a balance in your life,
acknowledge the great powers around us and in us.
If you can do that, and live that way, you are really wise.
- Euripides

The Perfect Balance Diet is based on the principle that everything is connected. When we are out of balance in one area of our lives, it shows up in other areas of our lives, too. We might not recognize it, or understand that the two things are related, but one thing affects the other nonetheless. We might attempt to "fix" the second thing, but if we don't fix the first thing, the thing that caused it to get out of balance in the first place, it will just come back again. And usually, we end up with so many little imbalances that we don't know which came first. We could spend years working on symptoms, but until we get to the cause, the root of the imbalance, then we're wasting our time.

So, how do we start? We start by looking at where we want to be. We remember what it looks like and feels like to be in balance, to be comfortable, and content, and healthy. And then we strive for that. We work to bring ourselves back into that state of perfect balance. It's not about losing anything. It's about gaining balance. It's about being in harmony with nature. When we look at nature as our guide, we don't see many overweight animals out in the wild. Can you imagine a giraffe, or a dolphin, or kangaroo hopping on a scale every day to check their weight, or putting themselves on a diet to lose weight? There's no need! These creatures follow their instincts. They know what to eat, when to eat, and how to eat. They know how to adapt to their surroundings. They know how to take care of themselves.

As humans, this should all be easy for us, right? But it's not. As time has gone on and we've evolved into this modern society, we have many, many more choices available to us than we have ever had. And some of those choices are not the best ones for us. With the added convenience of transportation we have learned to move less, so we're getting less exercise. With the advent of technology we are at our desks more, and getting less sunshine. Our foods can come to us ready-made to save time, and yet they're often frozen and microwavable which discounts many of the nutrients our bodies crave. We're a global society, so we can work odd hours yet doing so messes up our sleep cycle.

To get back into balance, we need to be reminded of our own true nature.

⌐⟪ AYURVEDA ⟫¬

Ayurveda, the "Science of Life" from India, dates back more than 5,000 years. The first written records of Ayurveda are found in the Vedas, the oldest and largest body of knowledge in history. But Ayurveda is even older than this, because it started as an oral tradition, with the knowledge being passed down by the rishis, who studied nature and its laws and how these laws relate to human beings.

Ayurvedic knowledge spread into other parts of the world as time went on. Eventually, it made its way to Greece, where it had a profound influence on the development of medicine there. Greek medicine later evolved into Allopathic medicine, which is the type of medicine most practiced today.

Fast forward to centuries later, when here in the west, we started learning about Ayurveda from the Maharishi Mahesh Yogi, Deepak Chopra, Vasant Lad and other scholars. Now we are lucky to have many fine schools where we can study Ayurveda in the U.S., including the Maharishi University of Management, the California College of Ayurveda and the Ayurvedic Institute. Ayurveda is a sister science to yoga and meditation, and they are best practiced together. Now that yoga is so prevalent in the west, people are embracing Ayurveda more and more.

According to Ayurveda, there are three operating principles of nature, or doshas, that we can call mind/body types. The doshas are made up of the five elements (air, space, fire, water, and earth). Since every one of us has all five of the elements in our physiology, we each have all three doshas as well, just in different proportions.

⊶ THE THREE DOSHAS ⊷

While we cannot see these doshas, we see the effect that they have on our mind and body. They operate as "metabolic principles." Each person is born with a unique combination of each of these three doshas, which make up his or her mind/body type. The goal is to find your particular mind/body type and keep it in balance for optimum health and happiness. This balance is achieved through diet, exercise, and lifestyle.

Our dosha is like our fingerprint, unique to us. We all have the three doshas in our physiology, just in different proportions. The idea is to find out which dosha is most dominant for you, and how you can strive to keep yourself in balance using the various recommendations for your dosha.

Vata is made up of air and space. Vata-type people are generally thin and find it hard to gain weight. Because of this, Vatas have very little energy reserve and can tire easily when they overextend themselves which them gets them out of balance. Vatas need to get sufficient rest and not overdo things, stay warm, and keep a regular lifestyle routine. The hummingbird is an example of Vata in nature.

Pitta is made up of fire and water. Pitta-type people are generally of medium size and well proportioned. They have a medium amount of physical energy and stamina. They also tend to be intelligent and have a sharp wit and a good ability to concentrate. The eagle is an expression of Pitta in nature.

Kapha is made up of earth and water. Kapha-type people tend to have sturdy, heavy frames, providing a good reserve of physical strength and stamina. This strength gives Kaphas a natural resistance to disease and a generally positive outlook about life. The swan is a very Kapha-like creature.

Here is a list of just some of the qualities that come along with each dosha. Take a look and see which dosha fits you the most. Because we each have all three doshas in our system, you might have two of the dosha come up equally. Many people are "double doshas" in which case you'll want to follow the routine for your dosha according to the seasons. For a most specific assessment, you may choose to consult an Ayurvedic practitioner, who will find your natural state of balance and current state of imbalance through traditional ayurvedic diagnostic tools such as pulse reading.

VATA
____ My hands and feet tend to be cold.
____ My skin tends to be dry.
____ My hair tends to be dry.
____ I like to be active, "on the go," I find it hard to sit still.
____ My appetite varies
____ I tend to eat quickly; I have a delicate digestion.
____ I get worn out easily.
____ I am fairly flexible, mentally and physically.
____ When conflicts arise I can be anxious and restless.
____ My moods change quickly.

PITTA
____ My hands and feet are usually warm.
____ My skin is soft and ruddy, or freckled.
____ My hair is fine, thin, reddish, or prematurely gray.
____ I enjoy physical activities with a purpose, especially competitive ones.
____ I feel uncomfortable skipping meals.
____ I have a strong digestion; I can eat almost anything.
____ I am fairly strong and can handle various physical activities.
____ I am fairly muscular.
____ When conflicts arrive, I can become intense and irritable.
____ My moods change slowly, but I can snap when agitated.

KAPHA
____ My hands are usually cool.
____ My skin is oily and moist.
____ My hair is thick and wavy.
____ I like leisurely activities best.
____ I like to eat but can skip meals easily.
____ I eat and digest slowly.
____ I have good stamina and a steady energy level.
____ I am fairly solid and big-boned.
____ When conflicts arise, I can get lazy or depressed.
____ My moods are mostly steady, I'm pretty easy-going.

TOTAL: _____ VATA   _____ PITTA   ____ KAPHA

Being in balance not only means being healthier and happier, but also being the best person you can be. Here are some of the character traits of doshas when they are in balance versus when they are out of balance:

	VATA	PITTA	KAPHA
When in Balance You Are:	- Enthusiastic - Alert - Flexible - Creative - Talkative - Responsive	- Loving - Content - Intelligent - Articulate - Courageous	- Affectionate - Steady - Methodical - High stamina - Resistant to illnesses
When Out of Balance You Are:	- Restless - Fatigued - Constipated - Anxious	- Perfectionist - Frustrated - Angry - Impatient - Irritable - Prematurely gray or have early hair loss	- Dull - Prone to oily skin - Prone to allergies - Possessive - Oversleeping

To get an idea about what the doshas look like here are some examples of celebrities and their dominant doshas:

VATA:
Barack Obama, Megan Fox, Jim Carrey, Uma Thurman, Steven Spielberg, Celine Dion, Ashton Kutcher

PITTA:
Madonna, Donald Trump, Julianne Moore, Brad Pitt, Jennifer Aniston, Hillary Clinton, Katie Couric

KAPHA:
George Clooney, Jennifer Lopez, Oprah Winfrey, Placido Domingo, Angelina Jolie, Deepak Chopra, Beyoncé

⌁❦ SEASONAL RECOMMENDATIONS ❦⌁

Weather and seasonal changes affect our balance. Everyone can benefit from adapting his or her routine to the season. November through February in the Northern Hemisphere, when it is cold and dry, is Vata season. When wind, cold, and dry weather continues, Vata accumulates in the environment, which can cause a Vata imbalance in the body. During this season, it is a good idea to adopt a more Vata diet and routine to keep Vata in balance. Stay warm, eat warm foods, and don't wear yourself out. To stay in harmony with nature, eat foods that are fresh during these months, like apples, pears, broccoli, endive, kale, pomegranates, pumpkins, and Brussels sprouts.

Pitta season comes during the summer, July through October in the Northern Hemisphere, when the weather is hot. To keep Pitta in balance during this time, eat cool foods, such as salads. Drink cool, not ice cold, liquids, and avoid too much sun. Melons, berries, corn, cucumber, peaches, squash, and sweet peppers are all fresh and abundant during the summer season.

Springtime, March through June in the Northern Hemisphere, is Kapha season, when it is cold and wet. This is the time you are more likely to get a cold from a Kapha imbalance. Stay warm, eat light meals, and get enough regular exercise to help keep Kapha in balance. In the spring you'll find fresh snap peas, scallions, oranges, lettuce, cherries, grapefruit, and new potatoes.

	VATA	PITTA	KAPHA
Season:	Fall/Winter (Cold & Dry)	Summer (Hot)	Spring (Cold & Wet)

Just as we are influenced by the doshas during the seasons, we are influenced by each dosha as we age. There are seasons to our lives.

⌁❦ KAPHA ❦⌁

Childhood has all the qualities of Kapha. This "season" of our lives lasts from when we are born until about age 20 or so. As children, we are more Kapha-like. We may have a little bit of baby fat; we're more calm and carefree. We place an emphasis on friendship and love to be cuddled.

When we are children, it might take longer for us to learn things, but once we learn them, we never forget. It might have taken quite a while to learn the alphabet, to get all 26 letters in the right order. But I think we've all got it down now, even though we don't practice every day!

When we're very young, we take a lot of naps, and sleep long hours at a time. Then we go through another stage as teenagers where we sleep a lot, too. This is all very Kapha-like behavior.

Kids also tend to get a lot of colds, especially during the pre-school years. Colds and congestion are Kapha imbalances. Like increases like, and kids share their germs freely when they gather together on a regular basis. Kapha associated with Kapha produces more Kapha, and too much Kapha leads to imbalance. Getting kids on a Kapha balancing routine during these times helps to balance them out.

⊶ PITTA ⊷

Sometime around age 20 our Pitta nature starts taking over. We might be in college, or just entering the working world, and our ambition becomes important to us. We become more competitive, we want to get ahead. We start thinking about money, and wanting those luxury items like fast cars.

At this age we are very busy building our careers, we are super work-oriented. We're in the thinking and planning phase of our lives. We've got this fire burning inside us, so we're a little more aggressive in going after what we want. We can be impatient.

This is the time when we use our intellect more than any other. Whether we're studying for exams or learning about our chosen field, we are constantly thinking. We're also strategizing and positioning ourselves. We look at where we are and where we're going. We like being in control.

As a part of this planning stage, we're also looking for our lifetime partner. We're discerning in this process, sorting out our priorities. We have lots of choices to make, but we know what we want – or at least we think we do! Our sexual desire is at its peak.

◦◦ **VATA** ◦◦

Then at about age 40 Vata comes strongly into play, and we become more Vata-like as we grow older. We start noticing that we don't remember things as well. At this age, our attention is also divided between work, family, community and other responsibilities, so we naturally have more on our minds. As we get older, more of Vata's physical ailments present themselves, too. Our fertility decreases. We may begin to have digestive problems, and our hearing may get a little worse. All these things are the effects of more Vata present in our system. This is the time for us to adapt our diet and exercise programs to include more Vata foods and activities.

Sometime after age 60 we may become more Kapha-like again. We slow down and want to surround ourselves with family. We're more concerned with comfort. It may be more difficult to stimulate our-selves physically to keep in balance, but we can certainly stimulate ourselves mentally, by taking classes and learning new things. We can continue to do things that we enjoy and engage in conversations with people we respect.

CHAPTER 2

FOOD
IT'S NOT JUST WHAT YOU EAT

Health is the greatest gift,
contentment the greatest wealth,
faithfulness the best relationship.
-Buddha

Food plays a big role in the Ayurvedic lifestyle. There is an Ayurvedic proverb that says: "When diet is wrong, medicine is of no use. When diet is correct, medicine is of no need." Digestion is a very important component in Ayurveda. We're not just what we eat, we are predominantly what we digest. Ayurveda explains that there are three parts to the digestive process: digestion, assimilation, and elimination of food. When our digestion is efficient, the rest follows more easily, so we get the optimal benefit from our food. When our digestion is strong, our immune system is strong.

In Ayurveda, our digestive fire is called agni. When our agni is strong then our appetite is strong. To maintain healthy digestion, which helps us to digest our food and absorb the nutrients in our food, It's not just what we eat, it's also how we eat it. Ayurveda offers these suggestions:

⊷ EATING FOR OPTIMAL DIGESTION ⊷

‾It's always nice to set the table for a meal. Remove clutter and provide a calm atmosphere in which to eat.

‾Eat only when you are hungry. And eat before you get so hungry that you are uncomfortable. 3-5 hours between meals is usually best.

‾Stop eating when you feel about 75% full. Don't overstuff yourself. Eating too much food overloads your digestive system and can lead to a build-up of toxins. Ayurveda calls these toxins "ama" – it's a sticky waste product of digestion that clogs the channels of circulation in the body so that nutrients can't get to where they need to go. Ama in the body makes us feel heavy and dull. And over time, if we don't get rid of the ama, we may experience constipation or diarrhea, joint pain, or even a lowered immune system.

‾Sit down while eating, and pay attention to the meal that you are eating. Really taste the food, smell the food, take in the colors of the food. This helps to make the experience of eating more pleasant.

‾Don't watch TV or read while you are eating. And don't talk on the phone or drive while eating. All of these activities just serve as a distraction to the food that interrupts the digestive process and can cause you to overeat.

‾Make sure to include all six tastes (sweet, sour, salty, bitter, pungent, and astringent) in each meal so that you feel satisfied after you eat. Most of the time when we get those cravings after dinner, when we feel like we need "more" or we want to go back for second helpings, it's because we are lacking one or more of those six tastes. Including all of the six tastes keeps us satiated so that the meal itself is enough for us.

‾Avoid ice-cold food and beverages. Cold water douses the digestive fire. At a restaurant, ask for water without ice. Adding a slice of lemon is also beneficial in stimulating digestion. Lemon is warming, for Vatas and Kaphas. Lime is cooling, which is better for Pittas, and better during the hot summer months.

- Sit quietly for a few minutes after eating. Don't rush to your next activity. Spend some time being still and grateful for the meal.

A crust eaten in peace
is better than a banquet
partaken in anxiety.
-Aesop

◦❀ **ENERGY** ❀◦

Ayurveda explains that the foods we eat have a big influence on the amount of energy we have. We can be mindful in what we purchase, and what we choose to eat, to get the most energy from our foods.

- Fresh fruits and vegetables give us lots of energy right away. It is important for us to both cut and cook the vegetables ourselves for optimum energy. It may be convenient to buy pre-cut up veggies in the market, but those have already lost some of their prana, the vital energy that is in this produce and also in the air that we breathe.

- Avoid frozen, canned, processed or leftover foods. Foods that have been altered with artificial flavorings or preservatives are more difficult to digest. These foods can make us feel more fatigued. Chetana is a Sanskrit word meaning "nature's intelligence." Food that is fresh and wholesome is abundant with chetana, so it can provide us with the nutrients that our bodies need in an efficient manner. Once food has been processed, frozen, chemically enhanced, or microwaved it loses some of its chetana. Foods that are alive with chetana are more easily digested and assimilated into our bodies. Foods that lack chetana are more difficult to digest and can leave us feeling sluggish. When choosing which foods to eat, reach for foods that are as fresh, and freshly prepared as possible.

- Choose locally grown and organic foods, so the body doesn't have to work overtime to try to purify itself after eating. Most grocery stores now have an organic section in their produce departments. The term "organic" means that this is food that has been cultivated and processed without any chemicals. Since there is nothing to kill the bugs, and no wax on the apples, the fruits and vegetables might not look as picture perfect as we have become used to, but they actually taste wonderful! Organic farming is better for the land as well, as the runoff from fertilized fields feeds into rivers and oceans, potentially polluting the water and posing hazards to life in and around it. Organic methods are really getting back to basics, the way we farmed back before any of these chemicals were created. Organic methods build up the soil, creating stronger, more disease-free plants. Going organic is a great choice, both nutritionally and ecologically.

- Watch food combinations. Avoid foods that don't digest well in combination. For example, milk should only be consumed with sweet tastes, such as rice, wheat, or sugar. Milk should never be consumed with yogurt, eggs, or fish.

- Avoid caffeine, in soda, coffee or tea. Caffeine is energy draining in the long run; it taxes the liver, creating fatigue and a build up of toxins. Instead choose pure water, or herb teas, which help to flush toxins from the system.

- Choose restaurants carefully. When you cook at home, you know that you are using the freshest ingredients, and cooking with mindfulness and love. In restaurants, be aware of what ingredients are used as well as the cooking methods.

- Almonds, cashews and walnuts are excellent sources of protein, and are more digestible if they are soaked or cooked before eating.

- Eat a variety of foods, to satisfy all six tastes (sweet, sour, salty, bitter, pungent and astringent) and prevent food "boredom." This can be challenging given our western influences and the mostly sweet, sour and salty food available in American restaurants.

Man seeks to change the foods available in nature
to suit his tastes, thereby putting an end
to the very essence of life contained in them.
–Sai Baba

❧ BREAKFAST ❧
With our western penchant for busy-ness many of us skip break-fast, thinking we don't have time as we're rushing around in the morning. According to Ayurveda, we're doing ourselves a disservice. Fasting irritates all of the doshas, and missing breakfast is particularly bad for Pitta, making us irritable and unsettled as we start our day. What to do? Eat something!

Blended fresh fruit and/or vegetable juice is a great way to rehydrate the body after the night's fast. Citrus is too acidic for an empty stomach, so try alternatives like apple, pear, or grape. Fresh juice is best, and it should be served at room temperature or slightly cooled. Cooked apples are another wonderful way to start your day the ayurvedic way. Morning is the perfect time to get the maximum benefit from fruit. It helps with our digestion and overall well-being.

❧ LUNCH ❧
Digestion is affected not only by what we eat and how we eat, but also when we eat. Because our digestion is strongest midday, between the hours of noon and 1 pm, lunch should ideally be our largest meal of the day. We want to wait 3-5 hours in between meals to eat so that the digestive process is completed from the previous meal before we go ahead and put more food into our stomachs. It's okay to snack on some nuts or crackers and hummus in between meals if you feel like you need to keep your energy up. Just don't eat so much that your snack becomes a meal in itself.

❧ DINNER ❧
The best time for dinner is anywhere between 5:30 and 7 pm. It's a good idea to complete the meal before 7 pm so that the body has at least 3 hours before bedtime to adequately digest the food. When the food has been digested, the body can then focus on sleep. Since the ideal bedtime is 10 pm, the guideline is to finish dinner by 7 pm. A small snack or dessert is fine after dinner, but try not to eat anything after 8 pm.

❧ RAW FOODS ❧
There's a big trend now toward eating raw foods. I can understand the principle behind it, raw foods and juices are very cleansing and energizing, they contain a lot of natural intelligence. Sprouts have enzymes that help with digestion, and some of the spicier sprouts

help to eliminate toxins, which Ayurveda calls "ama". However, for the nutrients in food to be properly assimilated into the body, food must be cooked. Cooking happens either outside the body, the conventional way with heat in the kitchen, or food can be cooked in the stomach. The digestive fire has to be really strong to provide enough energy to cook the food inside the body. Pittas can handle eating raw foods, because they have a strong agni, or digestive fire. Kaphas can eat some raw foods, particularly during the summer, but they generally fare better with cooked foods. Raw foods are not good for Vatas. Because of their sensitive digestion, Vatas need to favor warm, cooked foods.

> *One should eat to live, not live to eat.*
> *–Moliere*

⟡ SNACKS ⟡

⟡ RAISINS ⟡
Raisins are balancing for Vata because they are sweet, and especially balancing for Pitta because they are also cooling. Because they are heavy to digest, and have a high glycemic index, raisins are best eaten in moderation. Cinnamon helps to lower the glycemic index, so adding a little cinnamon to raisins is a good idea. Raisins are found in many Indian dishes.

In Ayurveda, raisins are known to be very healing, and by using raisins in food, we reap the benefits simply by eating! The medicinal qualities of raisins are many. Raisins are lubricating to the body, especially the lungs. And raisins are good for both the brain, and the mind; they can help to uplift and balance emotions. Raisins with either milk or water are very good for relieving thirst. To help with bowel function, soak some raisins overnight and eat them and drink the raisin-water in the morning. Raisins have also been known to support fertility in women. It is best to store raisins in the refrigerator to prevent fermentation.

⟡ ALMONDS ⟡
Almonds are one of the best foods for pacifying Vata. They're sweet and warm, high in protein, and loaded with vitamin E and

magnesium. They're also a good source of calcium, iron, potassium and zinc. Because almonds are raw, and heavy, Ayurveda gives us some recommendations about how to eat them so that we can digest them more easily. It is a good idea to soak almonds in water overnight. Peeling the skin off of almonds also helps their digestibility. Almonds are best eaten with other foods, like grains or vegetables. I add sliced almonds to our salads, or sprinkle them on hot cereal. They're also really great added to breads and muffins. Eating almonds helps to balance Vata, and applying warm, sweet almond oil to the skin is a real treat. Almond oil is a wonderful massage oil for Vatas.

◦❀ FRUIT ❀◦

We all grow up knowing that fruit is an important food to include in our diet because it is whole and fresh and healthy. In Ayurveda, how and when we eat fruit is important to consider. Fruit should always be eaten on an empty stomach, or before a meal, because fruit goes through the digestive tract more quickly than other foods. When we eat fruit on an empty stomach it helps us to detoxify the body and supplies us with needed energy for weight loss and other activities. However, when we eat fruit after a meal, the fruit is prevented from digesting because it is being blocked by the other foods that are ahead of it in line. So the fruit juices come into contact with the other foods, turns into acid, and the whole meal starts to ferment and spoil. When fruit mixes with other foods, it produces gas, so we feel bloated and burpy.

Ayurveda says that eating whole fruit is preferable to drinking fruit juice. If you want to drink fruit juice, choose fresh fruit juice, never juice from a can. Don't drink juice that has been heated, as heating juice, or cooking fruit, takes away many of the nutrients. When drinking fruit juice, take sips to mix the juice with saliva for better digestion, don't take big gulps.

It is always best to choose fresh fruits that are in season. There are certain fruits that are more balancing for each dosha, so be sure to check the Dosha Diet charts in the weight management chapter.

◦❀ THE BASICS OF AYURVEDIC COOKING ❀◦

Ayurveda sees cooking as an important part of the whole digestion and nutrition process. Anyone can cook ayurvedically; we just need to follow a few simple guidelines. The taste that accompanies food gives information to the body, and every taste has a specific effect. A balanced meal in Ayurveda contains each of the six tastes: sweet, sour, salty, bitter, pungent, and astringent. Because fresh foods provide the maximum amount of energy, Ayurveda recommends that we use fresh foods while cooking. Avoid eating leftovers, and frozen or processed foods whenever possible, as they lack vital energy and are more difficult to digest. Vegetables are more efficiently digested and assimilated when they are cooked, so Ayurvedic cooking principles advise that we cook our veggies rather than eating them raw.

The environment comes into play when cooking, too. To help our bodies acclimate and stay in balance, Ayurveda recommends that we seasonally favor dosha balancing foods in each of the three seasons, Vata (Fall/Winter), Pitta (Summer), and Kapha (Spring). And cook with love in your heart, so that positive emotions infuse your meals.

⊶ **RICE** ⊷

Rice is used in India for many different ceremonies. It is used in offerings, and colored, powdered rice is used to create mandalas. Rice is a symbol of health and wealth in many countries. We often toss rice at newlyweds to wish them fertility and prosperity. There are many different kinds of rice, including brown, wild, jasmine, Arborio and Basmati. The white rices are considered more easily digestible. Of all the rices, Ayurveda favors Basmati, because it balances all three of the doshas. And Ayurveda says that we need to avoid rice that is instant, pre-cooked, or leftover because it has less nutrition and life energy in it.

And here's a tip: Ayurveda says to only add salt to the rice after it is cooked, because adding the salt to the cooking water can affect the cooking temperature of the rice. Rice can be used so many ways, and cooked with spices, nuts, vegetables or beans. When sweetened with milk rice can also be made into a delicious dessert. Ayurveda suggests that we eat rice several times during the week, but not everyday. It is a good idea to alternate the rice in our meals with other grains such as couscous, quinoa, and barley.

I love to cook comfort food. I'll make fish and vegetables
or meat and vegetables and potatoes or rice.
The ritual of it is fun for me, and the creativity of it.
−Reese Witherspoon

⟨⟨ **GHEE** ⟩⟩

Ghee is clarified butter, and the preferred oil to cook with in Ayurveda. Oil is seen as a carrier, helping the body to absorb and assimilate the nutrients in food. We have delicious organic ghee at DharmaSmart.com, or you can buy ghee in most health food stores.

To make your own ghee at home, put one pound of unsalted butter into a saucepan and heat slowly until completely melted. Turn the heat down to low. The melted butter appears cloudy, and at first a white foam rises to the top. The foam then falls to the bottom as the melted butter starts to clear, and the sediment is more visible at the bottom. Simmer until the sediment becomes golden brown and the rest of the liquid becomes clear and golden. At this point it kind of smells like popcorn! Remove from heat and cool for 10 minutes. Line a strainer with cheesecloth or muslin and place over a glass jar. Pour the ghee through the strainer, taking care not to pour in any of the sediment. As the ghee cools it will solidify. It does not need to be refrigerated.

⟨⟨ **OLIVE OIL** ⟩⟩

Olive oil is nothing short of amazing. It offers all of the benefits of the olive fruit, including the vitamins, flavor, and aroma. Olive oil is used in massage because it is readily absorbed into the skin. Research has shown that olive oil is good for our health, too, in that it can lower the incidence of gallstones, and may help prevent color cancer. A recent study from the University Hospital of Valme in Seville, Spain, showed that olive oil has some strong antibacterial properties, which could be helpful in preventing peptic ulcers or even stomach cancer. Olive oil should be stored in a cool, dark place to keep it fresh. Here's an explanation of the different varieties of olive oil:

- Extra virgin: considered the best, least processed, from the first pressing of the olives.

- Virgin: from the second pressing.

- Pure: undergoes some processing, such as filtering and refining.

- Extra light: undergoes considerable processing and retains a very mild olive flavor.

❧ GARLIC ❧

Garlic has powerful anti-viral properties. Ayurveda has known this for centuries! Many people who use garlic on a regular basis claim that they have immunity from any cold and flu viruses. There are garlic capsules available now, and the upside is that you don't get the odor associated with this bulbous plant. But there is no substitute for the real thing. Garlic is a favorite in many ethnic recipes, and for good reason – it's delicious! Garlic also stimulates digestion and helps with overall rejuvenation. Garlic can be added to sauces, or salads, or you can bake the cloves whole and use them as a delicious spread on crackers or bread.

I always say centered food
equals centered behavior.
–Marilu Henner

❧ SPICES ❧

❧ GINGER ❧

Ginger is used often in Ayurvedic cooking. It can be used in so many ways, both fresh and dried. Fresh ginger is balancing for both Vata and Pitta. Dried ginger, because it is stronger and more concentrated, is balancing for Kapha. Ginger kindles agni, the digestive fire, so it helps the body to digest, absorb and assimilate food. Ginger is especially helpful in the cold winter months. It makes food lighter and easier and more digestible. It is also wonderful to help alleviate coughs, congestion and runny noses.

❧ GARAM MASALA ❧

Garam Masala, found on spice racks and in recipes, is not a spice in itself, but a blend of spices used throughout India. Garam means "hot" and Masala means "spice." The spices, and some of the proportions in Garam Masala can vary depending on personal taste, and the region. Here's a sample recipe so that you can make your own Garam Masala at home. This recipe makes about ½ cup of Garam Masala, and when kept in an airtight container will stay fresh for 3 months. I've seen different recipes that use mace and/or fenugreek, so experiment and see what you like.

- ⁻2 Tablespoons cumin seeds
- ⁻2 Tablespoons coriander seeds
- ⁻2 Tablespoons cardamom seeds
- ⁻2 Tablespoons black peppercorns
- ⁻1 3" stick cinnamon, broken up
- ⁻1 teaspoon whole cloves
- ⁻1 teaspoon grated nutmeg
- ⁻1/2 teaspoon saffron (optional)

Put all of the spices except the nutmeg and saffron in a dry, heavy skillet over medium-high heat. Toast the spices about 10 minutes, stirring occasionally, until they turn several shades darker and give off a sweet, smoky aroma. Let cool completely. Transfer the spice mixture to a spice mill or coffee grinder and grind to a powder. Stir in the nutmeg and saffron.

> *You can easily put together your own favorite spice blend,*
> *whether that's a salt and pepper mixture or you're adding herbs*
> *to it or Creole spice. Just watch out for the sodium content.*
> *That why I encourage you to make your own.*
> *–Emeril Lagasse*

◦⚛ **TURMERIC** ⚛◦

Turmeric is known to support important blood and liver functions, and to be an abundant source of healthful antioxidants. Many women in India credit their beautiful skin, hair, and nails, to a diet rich in Turmeric. Turmeric has the tastes of pungent, bitter, and astringent. These tastes are difficult to find in the typical western diet, and they are essential for balancing the Kapha dosha.

Ayurvedic physicians have used as turmeric in healing compounds for centuries, and western medicine is just starting to catch on to its many benefits now. "Cancer Research" published a study, which shows that turmeric, and its active ingredient, curcumin, may have the ability to treat and even prevent prostate cancer when combined with a certain group of vegetables like broccoli, kale, Brussels sprouts, cauliflower or cabbage. Interesting to note that while prostate cancer is a definite concern for American men, it barely affects Indian men.
Turmeric is one of the oldest, most important spices in ayurvedic cooking.

It is the spice that gives curry its yellow color. Due to its heating quality, turmeric helps to balance Kapha and Vata doshas and because it also has a bitter taste, it helps to balance the Pitta dosha, thus making it tri-doshic. Turmeric is also beneficial for helping with occasional congestion, and soothing a hoarse voice or the occasional cough.

Curry is actually a blend of herbs that is abundant in Indian cooking.

If you're interested in making your own curry blend, experiment to see how spicy you like it. Red pepper, black pepper, mustard seed and chili flakes are optional. I like a very mild curry, so this is a combination that works for me. Mix together:

- 1/2 teaspoon ground ginger
- 1 teaspoon ground cumin
- 1 teaspoon ground coriander
- 2 teaspoons ground turmeric

⊳※ CUMIN ※⊲

Cumin is popular in Indian, Mexican and Middle Eastern cuisines. According to Ayurveda, it is balancing for all three doshas. It has been known to aid digestion and help flush toxins out of the body.

Cumin can be used either as whole seeds or ground, raw or dry-roasted. Ground raw, it is a dull brown color, which is enriched by being sautéed in Ghee or oil. Powdered dry-roasted cumin is a rich brown in color. Both sautéing and roasting make the aroma and flavor of cumin come alive. Cumin combines well with a wide range of other spices, including turmeric, fennel, coriander, ginger and cinnamon. Cumin is especially delicious in dahl and soups.

⊳※ CORIANDER ※⊲

Coriander is a tridoshic spice much revered in ayurveda. It is a cooling spice and contributes the sweet and astringent tastes. Ayurvedic texts suggest that it is good for digestion, whets the appetite, helps combat allergies and also helps purify the blood. Coriander by itself has a sharp aroma and smells and tastes best freshly ground in a coffee or spice mill.

Ground coriander can be added along with other spices to dahls and vegetables as you cook.

⊶ FENNEL ⊷

At Indian restaurants you may see fennel seeds instead of after dinner mints. This is because fennel is extremely good for the digestion. It acts as a general toner for the digestive system, and is particularly good for enhancing Agni, the digestive fire, without aggravating Pitta. In India, eating a few toasted fennel seeds after a meal is a common practice, and it is also used to freshen the breath. Fennel has a distinctive smell rather like Aniseed, or licorice. It has a nutty flavor and a strong aroma when sautéed in Ghee. Fennel is considered a cooling spice, and it has the taste of both sweet and bitter.

⊶ BASIL ⊷

Sweet Basil is used in cooking in both its fresh and dried forms. Basil is balancing for Vata and Kapha and for Pitta when used in lesser quantities. It is a warming herb, and contributes the sweet, bitter and pungent tastes. Basil is easy to grow outdoors in the summer months, and I love to have some on hand right in my backyard for whenever I want to make bruschetta or add some fresh basil to sauces or salads.

Basil can also be made into a tea, and this is often used in ayurveda to maintain and promote the long-term health of the respiratory tract. It is also used to settle stomach disorders and to enhance digestion. A mild natural sleep aid, Basil enhances the quality of sleep. Dried basil is aromatic and is wonderful to flavor soups and stews. It is stronger in flavor when dried, so you don't need very much of it.

⊶ CINNAMON ⊷

Cinnamon is the peeled bark of an evergreen tree. There are many different types of cinnamon found throughout the world. The kind we find most often in the U.S. is from the cassia tree, and is harvested in Vietnam, Indonesia and China. The characteristic spicy flavor of cinnamon comes from its essential oils. These oils are what gives cinnamon it's healthful benefits, too. Cinnamon tea can freshen breath, and relieve an upset stomach. The fragrance of cinnamon can scent an entire room! I like to boil cinnamon sticks right on the kitchen stove to get that warm, homey feeling going.

Cinnamon is a warming spice, and is consists of sweet, pungent and bitter tastes. It is excellent for pacifying Kapha and good for

balancing Vata also. In ayurveda, cinnamon is used to assist digestion and to calm stomach disorders. Studies have shown that just
half a teaspoon of cinnamon a day could reduce total cholesterol by
12 to 30 percent, while it also boosts the body's ability to store blood
sugar. You can add a sprinkle of cinnamon to your morning oatmeal,
on your toast, or in your hot cocoa. You can also sprinkle some
cinnamon in chili, or on sweet potatoes, or add it to baked goods.

✐❀ BLACK PEPPER ❀✐

Black pepper is widely used as a seasoning in the Western world.
In ayurvedic cooking, black pepper in all its forms: peppercorns,
cracked pepper and ground black pepper, is used as well. Pepper
has cleansing and antioxidant properties, and it is a bioavailability
enhancer, meaning that it helps to transport the benefits of any
other herbs to the different parts of the body. Pepper also helps
the free flow of oxygen to the brain, helps enhance digestion and
circulation, stimulates the appetite, and helps maintain respiratory
system health and the health of the joints.

Black pepper is a warming spice and has a pungent taste. It is terrific for pacifying Kapha, and just a little bit helps pacify Vata.
Black pepper should be used in moderation as it does increase Pitta.

✐❀ MINT ❀✐

Mint is a hearty plant and easy to grow. I've got an abundance of
two different kinds in my front yard! There are many varieties of
mint, including the popular Spearmint and Peppermint. Mint is a
cooling herb, with a sweet taste and a pungent after taste. Most
varieties of mint are pacifying for all three doshas, and since it is
cooling, mint is especially helpful for balancing Pitta. Mint is good
for the digestion as well as for respiratory system health. You can
make a tea out of dried mint for a refreshing summer beverage.
Mint is also delicious added to chutney.

✐❀ CARDAMOM ❀✐

Cardamom is often used in desserts in India and the Middle East. It is
considered a warming spice, and it has both sweet and pungent tastes.
Cardamom is considered tridoshic, balancing to all three doshas – however Pittas need to use smaller amounts of any pungent spice. Cardamom
is really good to help with digestions. It can help reduce bloating and gas.

You can chew up cardamom seeds to freshen the breath, and ease a sore throat. This is a really good tip that I got from Dr. Vasant Lad, one of the world renowned authorities on Ayurveda. He offered me some cardamom seeds on a break during one of his lectures. Delicious!

◦⊷ CHURNAS ⊶◦

According to Ayurveda, a balanced diet contains all six tastes at every meal. This can be challenging given our western influences. And since we want to make sure that we are getting the right proportion of flavors for our own dominant dosha, we tend not to want to overdo it. There's a simple solution! An herb and spice blend called a "Churna" that is specially formulated for Vata, Pitta or Kapha balancing. You can use this blend while cooking, or take the shaker with you to sprinkle on your food when you eat out. You can add it to sauces, soups, vegetable or rice dishes, even just sprinkle it on salads, popcorn or snacks. Very convenient, and really delicious. You can purchase a churna that is already made, such as those I have on my website DoshaSmart.com, or you can make your own blend at home with these recipes.

The Vata blend is calming, and includes cardamom, ginger, and other spices. The Pitta blend is cooling, and includes cumin, coriander and fennel along with other spices. The Kapha blend is invigorating, with turmeric, mustard, black pepper and more.

Vata Churna

INGREDIENTS:

- 2 tablespoons cumin seeds
- 2 tablespoons coriander seeds
- 1/2 teaspoon cardamom seeds
- 2 tablespoons fennel seeds
- 1 teaspoon ground ginger
- 1/4 teaspoon asafetida (hing powder)
- 1/4 teaspoon salt (I prefer Himalayan salt, it is unprocessed)
- 1 tablespoon raw sugar

INSTRUCTIONS:

In a dry skillet, roast the cumin and coriander seeds until nutty. Transfer to a spice grinder and add cardamom and fennel seeds; process to a fine powder. Put the ground spices in a bowl with the ground ginger, asafetida, and salt and mix all together. Transfer into a shaker bottle to use whenever you'd like.

Pitta Churna

INGREDIENTS:

- 2 tablespoons fennel seeds
- 2 tablespoons coriander seeds
- 2 tablespoons cumin seeds
- 1 tablespoon turmeric
- 2 tablespoons fresh mint leaves (chopped), or dried mint leaves
- 1/2 teaspoon ground ginger
- 1 tablespoon raw sugar

INSTRUCTIONS:

In a dry skillet, roast the coriander and cumin seeds until nutty. Transfer to a spice grinder and add the cardamom and fennel seeds; process to a fine powder. Put the spices in a bowl with the turmeric, mint, ground ginger and sugar and mix all together. Transfer into a shaker bottle to use whenever you'd like.

Kapha Churna

INGREDIENTS:

- 2 tablespoons coriander seeds
- 1 tablespoon cumin seeds
- 1 tablespoon fenugreek seeds
- 1 tablespoon ground ginger
- 1 tablespoon turmeric
- 1 tablespoon cinnamon
- 1 teaspoon ground clove
- 1/2 teaspoon black pepper

INSTRUCTIONS:

In a dry skillet, roast the coriander and cumin seeds until nutty. Transfer to a spice grinder and add the fenugreek seeds; process to a fine powder. Put the spices in a bowl with the ginger, turmeric, cinnamon, clove and black pepper and mix all together. Transfer into a shaker bottle to use whenever you'd like.

⊶⊸ **TEA** ⊷⊷

*Sometimes I get up very early in the morning
and enjoy a quiet house and cup of tea
before the craziness begins. Other times, I'll take a quick walk
on the beach. You can find peace in a few minutes.
—Cindy Crawford*

Green tea is known throughout the world for its medicinal properties. It's the abundance of antioxidants in the tea leaves that make it so beneficial. Antioxidants slow or prevent the oxidation of other molecules. Oxidation reactions in molecules can create free radicals that can turn into disease. Antioxidants are also important to overall cell health. Healthy cells mean less chance of disease. So antioxidants are an important part of preventive health care. Green tea is known to reduce the negative effects of "bad cholesterol"(LDL) by making more "good cholesterol" (HDL).

Green tea is also being studied as a preventative for Alzheimer's disease. Green tea has been known to prevent kidney stones, and it also helps keep bones strong, which fends off osteoporosis. Green tea gives fat metabolism a boost and its main antioxidant may even prevent cavities! Green tea has less caffeine than black tea, which has lots less caffeine than coffee, but if you want to make sure you avoid that stimulant altogether then reach for a decaffeinated variety of tea. Many brands also have green teas flavored with peach, orange or even mango!

Chai means "tea". Some stories say that Chai was invented by a royal king in the ancient courts of India and Siam who protected the recipe as one of his treasures. However, its roots can be traced unmistakably to Ayurveda. Chai is a traditional Indian drink, spicy and robust in flavor to stimulate the senses and soothe the soul. Served hot, with milk (I like to add vanilla soy milk) and sweetener, Chai is a wonderful treat in the winter months.

I absolutely love Chai, but as a Vata, I really can't have caffeine, so most of the time I end up making it myself rather than using tea bags, and that way I can make it decaf by starting with decaf black tea. The added benefit of making Chai at home is that you can add spices that are particularly balancing for your dosha, or you can make a tridoshic blend that is good for everyone! Herbs that are traditionally in Chai tea include:

- Cardamom

- Cinnamon

- Clove

- Black Pepper

- Ginger

- Fennel

Here are my suggestions for dosha-balancing Chai, to help get you started brewing up your personal blend:

- The Vata Blend: Ginger, cardamom, cinnamon.

- The Pitta Blend: Cardamom, cinnamon, fennel.

- The Kapha Blend: Ginger, Cardamom, cinnamon, cloves, black pepper.

- Tridoshic Blend: Cardamom, cinnamon, cloves, fennel, ginger.

Herb tea isn't actually "tea" made from tea leaves, it is an infusion made of herbs, greens, flowers or roots. Herb teas have been used as medicines for centuries. Here are some of the most popular herbal teas and their uses:

- Angelica Tea helps with both cough and colic.

- Chamomile Tea soothes the stomach and aids in relaxation.

- Ginseng Tea helps reduce fatigue, stress, and high blood pressure.

- Lemon Verbena Tea helps to bring down a fever, and also induces a restful sleep.

- Peppermint tea works wonders for nausea.

- Rose Hips tea is high in vitamin C and is good for fighting colds.

To me, the smell of fresh-made coffee
is one of the greatest inventions.
– Hugh Jackman

❧⬧ COFFEE ⬧❧

Because coffee contains caffeine, and Ayurveda tells us to avoid caffeine, Ayurveda does not recommend coffee. And for some people, especially Pittas, coffee is too acidic and can upset the stomach. However, coffee is considered to have the bitter taste that we lack in so many of our western foods, and that one reason why we crave it. If you choose to have coffee, go with the decaffeinated variety. You can also add herbs and spices to your coffee to make it more ayurvedic. Simply put your choice of herbs and spices on top of the coffee grounds before you run water through your drip coffee maker. The results will surprise you!

There are some good coffee substitutes, and most are made with grains. Teecino is a popular brand with lots of flavors. In ancient India, the kings, or "rajas" drank a nourishing ayurvedic beverage for strength and overall well-being. Now you can have it, too – it's called Raja's Cup! Raja's Cup tastes and smells just like coffee, but it is actually a precise blend of four potent herbs: Clearing Nut, Kasmard, Licorice and Winter Cherry — the combination of which helps to promote well-being and vitality. You can make it in your coffee maker just like you would regular coffee, or you can get the "tea bag" style where you just need to add hot water and you're good to go. You can find Raja's Cup on my DharmaSmart.com website.

CHAPTER 3

SLEEP AND RELATIONSHIPS
THE OTHER TWO PILLARS OF HEALTH

A well-spent day brings happy sleep.
– Leonardo da Vinci

Food, sleep, and relationships are the three pillars of health in Ayurveda. They are equally important to our overall feeling of well-being. They are like the three legs on a three-legged stool. If one leg is shorter than the others, then the whole stool is out of balance, there is no firm foundation to stand on. We need to pay attention to all three of these pillars of health to stay in Perfect Balance.

How well we sleep at night definitely has an effect on how well we function during the day. And it's not just the quantity of sleep we get; it's also the quality of sleep we get.

If you're having trouble getting to sleep, or if you're waking up and can't get back to sleep in the middle of the night, take a look at your environment, and see what changes need to be made. The Better Sleep Council (BetterSleep.org) has these tips to turn your bedroom into a sleep sanctuary:

- Keep a regular sleep routine. Head to bed at the same time each night to help program your body for sleep. Have some transition time between activity and sleep. Take a warm bath, or read an entertaining book.

- Keep your bedroom technology free. Many people keep a television in the bedroom, thinking this will help them relax or fall asleep at the end of the day. But television actually stimulates the mind, rather than settling it down. Even the most relaxing show interferes with our body clock because of the flickering lights. The same is true for the computer screen, or the cell phone.

- Don't bring work to bed with you. If you associate your bed with work, it is harder to wind down at night. Reserve your bed for sleep and sex only. That way, when you tuck yourself in, your body gets a powerful cue – it's time to sleep!

- Keep the bedroom dark and cool. In keeping with the cycle of nature, darkness triggers the body to produce melatonin, which helps us to sleep. Having too much light in the room confuses your body clock. If you don't have heavy curtains to block any outside light, try using a sleep mask. The temperature in the room also affects how well you sleep. Most people sleep best in a slightly cool room, not too hot or too cold.

- Make sure your bed is comfortable. You want your bed to be big enough so that you have enough room to stretch and turn comfortably. And if there are two of you that share a bed, you both need to have enough space. A Queen or King sized bed is best. If you're waking up with back pain, or you find that you are tossing and turning at night, check your bed for signs of wear, like lumps or sags. If you've had your mattress for five years or more, it might be time to get a new one.

- Your bed linens and pajamas should be soft and comfortable as well. Choose natural fabrics that feel good on your skin. Ayurveda says that 100% organic cotton is best because it allows your skin to breathe.

- Keep the room quiet. Sleep studies show that we get a more restful night's sleep when we are not distracted by sounds. If you can't avoid or eliminate noise from dogs, neighbors, or traffic, try masking it with a fan, with white noise, or with soothing music. Earplugs can also help.

- Invite sleep with fragrance. Aromatherapy helps to quiet the chatter in your mind. Essential oils in lavender, chamomile or sandalwood are particularly relaxing. Just a drop on your pillowcase will help you drift off into slumber.

When you create a sleep sanctuary you look forward to going to bed knowing that you are going to get a great night's sleep. Sweet dreams!

> *Think in the morning. Act in the noon.*
> *Eat in the evening. Sleep in the night.*
> *—William Blake*

⊶ THE DOSHAS AND SLEEP ⊷

Depending on your mind/body type, you may want to customize your sleep routine. Vatas get worn out easily, and need lots of sleep to renew themselves after a long day. Vatas do best on 9-10 hours of sleep a night. Yet, because the Vata mind is so restless, Vatas often have difficulty getting to sleep at night. One solution is to take a warm bath and allow enough time to settle down before bedtime.

Pittas need an average amount of sleep, 7-8 hours is fine. When Pitta has difficulty sleeping it is because they are thinking of work. It's a good idea for Pittas to take a cool shower, and relax before bedtime.

Kaphas have a large reserve of energy and do not require as much sleep. They can get by on 6-7 hours of sleep a night. Kaphas tend to sleep soundly, and they may have trouble waking up! Set the alarm to some uplifting music to help get the day started for sleepy Kaphas.

Ayurveda says that it is best for everyone to get to bed by 10 pm in keeping with the cycles of nature. That can be difficult for us, given that some great TV shows start at 10 pm, and we're often catching up on e-mail at that time! But Ayurveda has some very compelling reasons why 10 pm is the ideal bedtime, and these might inspire you to get to bed a little earlier from now on. First of all, 10 pm is the start of Pitta time. If we are already in bed sleeping, the body generates heat that can burn up any accumulated toxins. Sleep comes easier during Kapha time, which ends at 10 pm, because Kapha has the quality of slowness, and dullness, which helps us to relax into that sleep state. Pitta time is more stimulating, and we might even get the munchies as the time gets closer to midnight.

A ruffled mind makes a restless pillow.
-Charlotte Brontë

Another reason to get to bed earlier rather than later is that there is a solar energy that the earth retains up until midnight. The sleep we experience while this solar energy is in the atmosphere is very rejuvenating. It is powerfully beneficial for our health. Another way we can tell that the cycle of nature is conducive to sleep before 10 pm is the sounds we hear outside. Before 10 pm, we can hear the crickets singing in a soft melodic tone, a kind of Kapha lullaby. After 10 pm it turns into a much more sharp and piercing sound, indicative of Pitta.

From 10 pm to 2 am, this is the Pitta time when the body can get the rest it needs to restore energy and heal itself. We don't want to rob ourselves of this time. The hours from 2 am to 6 am are Vata time, when we dream. Our subconscious is solving problems for us, and working out events of the day. Then, in keeping with the harmony of nature, 6 am is the ideal time for us to wake up, with the sun as it is rising to start the day.

Our sleep affects our health and our general mood throughout the day. If you're tossing and turning, are restless, snore, or feel sleepy during the day, then you may be having problems getting the deep sleep you need. There are basically three different kinds of sleep disorders, one for each dosha. When you have trouble falling asleep, that is typically because of too much Vata. If you fall asleep, and then wake up in the middle of then night and can't get back to sleep, that is indicative of a Pitta imbalance. When you can't seem to get enough sleep, you have trouble waking up in the morning, then that shows an overabundance of Kapha. There are lots of reasons why we may have trouble sleeping, and no matter what they are, Ayurveda has these solutions to help us get that good night's rest:

- Avoid caffeine, especially after noon.

- Eat a light meal between 5 and 7 pm. This will give you time to digest before you go to sleep, so that you body can rest more soundly.

- An hour before bed, relax. Avoid stimulating activities such as working on the computer, or watching the nightly news. Take a nice bath, or listen to music. Use this time to wind down. Take slow, deep breaths.

- Get to bed by 10 pm. This is still Kapha time, when our body naturally wants to rest.

- Wear comfortable clothing to bed, breathable fabrics like cotton.

- Keep the room dark or dimly lit.

> *Man is a genius when he is dreaming.*
> *–Akira Kurosawa*

⊶ SNORING ⊷

About 45% of adults snore occasionally, and 25% snore on a regular basis. Problem snoring is more common in men, people who are overweight, and snoring can get worse as we get older. Snoring can affect our health, because we don't sleep as well at night. At it can also affect our relationships, because many couples can't even sleep in the same room at night because of snoring. But there are some ways that we can stop snoring. Here are some tips from the American Academy of Otolaryngology and the Minnesota Regional Sleep Disorders Center:

- Change your sleep position. Snoring most often occurs when you are lying on your back. In this position the tongue falls towards the throat. When you sleep on your side, air gets through more easily.

- Lose 10% of your body weight. Bulky neck tissue, which comes with excess weight, increases snoring. Even a modest weight loss will help with this.

- Avoid alcohol and sedatives. Both alcohol and sedatives such a sleeping pills can inhibit breathing and lead to snoring.

- Use steam before bed. Nasal congestion is a big cause of snoring. To reduce congestion inhale some steam, or take a steam shower.

- Try nasal strips. Over the counter nasal strips have been found to provide some relief from congestion and may also help prevent snoring.

If you have a severe snoring problem this may indicate a condition called sleep apnea where you could stop breathing. If none of these remedies work for you, consult with a sleep specialist for a proper evaluation and treatment options.

◦⊷ RELATIONSHIPS ⊶◦

> *Every person, all the events of your life are there*
> *because you have drawn them there.*
> *What you choose to do with them is up to you.*
> *-Richard Bach*

I have discovered a natural law that I call The Law of Relationship. It is two-fold, and it says 1) We are all connected. And 2) We are here to help each other learn and grow. If we keep this in mind at all times, all of our relationships will be more harmonious, more loving, and more fruitful.

Ayurveda is "The Science of Life." And life is all about relationships. It's about our relationship with our selves, our environment and all the people in our lives. Ayurveda can teach us how to get along with anyone, anytime, anywhere, because when we understand the principles behind this science, we are more understanding and accepting of a person's nature. We become better people because we learn to love "what is", rather than what we think "should be."

According to Ayurvedic wisdom, there are four basic principles of life. These principles are discussed in the Upanishads, the sacred texts from India. These principles form the foundation of Ayurveda, and they help us to understand the role that relationships play in our lives.

There is an organizing principle in the universe.
- This means that even though things might seem to be "random" there is a plan in play. There are no accidents, and there are no coincidences. Everything happens for a reason. We meet the people we meet for a reason. When we are aware of this, we can ask ourselves questions like: What can I learn from this person? How can I help this person?

Everything that exists is living.
Everything (yes, everything!) and everyone is made up of material (prakriti) and spirit (parusha). We vibrate with the life spirit that is in us and all around us. A relationship is a living thing as well; it has a life of its own. Relationships don't die, but they can, and do, change over time. We can ask ourselves what lessons we have to learn from a particular relationship, and how we can learn and grow from the experiences of a relationship, whatever they may be.

All existence is interconnected.
Everything and everyone in the universe is connected. Every pebble, every person, every bird, every rainbow, is connected to every other thing in one way or another. There is no separation between us. When we understand this, we know that any harm we do to another person, or thing, we are really doing to ourselves. This can help us to become more compassionate and loving people. We learn to take care of ourselves, of our relationships, of each other, and of the planet that we all share.

The essence of everything is a part of That – The Divine Creative Force.
Just as we are connected to each other, we are each also connected to the Whole, All That There Is, the Universe, God, Spirit, or whatever words you choose to use to describe that Divine Universal Energy that flows through us. Every action we take has repercussions that resonate out into the world. When we are happy, and living live "in love" then that love amps up the energy around us. It's contagious! We can't help but bring those good feelings with us wherever we go for everyone to pick up on. Healthy relationships are essential to the health of the whole planet.

> *Each friend represents a world in us,*
> *a world possibly not born until they arrive,*
> *and it is only by this meeting that a new world is born.*
> *-Anais Nin*

☙ LOVING "AS IS" ❧

In a relationship, you have a chance to see each other's quirks and idiosyncrasies. And as you spend more time together, those same quirks that you thought were so charming in the beginning may start to get on your nerves. When you say something about it, or try to change something about your partner, it only makes things worse. Or if you don't say something, and just stew about it, resentment builds up. So what do you do? Here are some ideas:

- Remember that whatever you pay attention to increases. Instead of focusing on the things you don't like, or have a problem with, focus on all the things you love, those good qualities.

- Practice acceptance. When you switch off judgment and instead accept your partner "as is," then you grow closer, and more intimate.

- De-stress. Take a deep breath. Usually you'll find that what's really bothering you is not your partner but the stress you've built up throughout the day. Meditate together, stretch, take a walk. To remind myself of this I made a T-shirt that says: "Less Moaning, More Om-ing."

- Mind your manners. Remember that you love this person. Be kind. Be respectful. Say "please," and "thank you." Give hugs and say "I love you," often!

Having someone wonder where you are
when you don't come home at night
is a very old human need.
-Margaret Mead

❖❀ COOPERATION ❀❖

Research from the University of California, San Diego, and Harvard University, provides the first laboratory evidence that cooperative behavior actually spreads from person to person to person. When we benefit from kindness, we "pay it forward" by helping others, which in turn creates a flow of cooperation that influences many more. And it only takes a few individuals to make a difference. The study shows that cooperative behavior spreads three degrees of separation, and that the effects persist over time. It is interesting to note that during the research an evolution of cooperation was found to develop. Groups with altruists in them end up being more altruistic as a whole, and more likely to progress and survive than the more selfish groups. One of the researchers, Nicholas Christakis, says "The flow of good and desirable properties like ideas, love, and kindness is required for human social networks to endure, and, in turn, networks are required for such properties to spread. Humans form social networks because the benefits of a connected life outweigh the costs."

> *I really admire bees' sense of common responsibility...*
> *Although sometimes individual bees fight,*
> *basically there is a strong sense of unity and cooperation.*
> *We human beings are supposed to be much more advanced,*
> *but sometimes we lag behind even small insects.*
> *– The Dalai Lama*

◦◦ HUG IT OUT ◦◦

Most times, at least here in the U.S., when we go in for a hug we go towards the person's right cheek. Maybe this is because most of us are right handed, but it seems to be the norm. If you do the muscle testing after this hug, you'll find that your muscle is weaker, meaning your energy level is down. However, when we hug left cheek to left cheek instead, the muscle testing shows that we are stronger, or that our energy level is up. Why is this? When we hug on the right side, we're connecting liver to liver. Our liver is where we hold our anger, so we are actually sharing our anger with each other for a brief moment. That weakens our energy. On the other hand, when we hug left to left, we connect at our heart centers, where we hold our love. The heart is located pretty centrally, but because of the direction of the blood flow, we can heart the heartbeat most easily on the left side. So by connecting for that brief moment with a hug to the left, we are sharing our love from that place in our hearts. Try it, and see if you can feel the difference!

◦◦ COMMUNICATION ◦◦

Communication is key to the success of a relationship, and listening is half of that equation. Probably the most important thing we can do in a relationship is to listen to the other person. When we feel heard, and understood, we feel safe and cared for. Listening is active and sometimes we have to practice to learn how to really do it well. Here are some tips:

- Focus on the person speaking. Let that person talk while you hear what they have to say. Make eye contact, and give feedback with body language such as nodding your head when you agree or understand.

- Pay attention to what is being said. Try to understand before you speak. Look for the main points that the person is sharing, and observe the person's body language as they are speaking. This will give you clues as to how they feel about what they are saying.

- Ask questions. It shows the person that you care about what they are saying. Ask them to clarify any points that you don't understand.

- When appropriate, take notes. When you're in a meeting and will be asked to remember the information later, write down what you need to know. Think about how this information is relevant to you, and that will help you to remember it.

Trouble is part of your life,
and if you don't share it,
you don't give the person who loves you
enough chance to love you enough.
-Dinah Shore

◦⊰❖⊱ TRUTHFULNESS ❖⊱◦

As a relationship expert, people often ask me what the secret to a successful relationship is. Most experts would say that it is communication. But what good is communication if you're not being truthful with one another? The most important ingredient in any relationship, whether it is a partnership, a friendship, or a marriage, is truthfulness. We need to take time to learn about the person we are with, and to also learn about ourselves and what we can contribute to a healthy relationship. Truthfulness is the foundation from which a relationship can grow. We need to be honest in every way, and about every thing. Without truth there can be no intimacy. Truth starts with being honest with ourselves.

Three things cannot be long hidden:
the sun, the moon, and the truth.
–Buddha

CHAPTER 4

HOUSE, HOME, HAVEN

Mid pleasures and palaces though we may roam,
Be it ever so humble, there's no place like home.
-John Howard Payne

Our physical environment is an extension of ourselves. Our energy affects the space, and the space affects our energy – and in turn, our health.

Have you ever noticed how there are some spaces you can walk into and immediately feel at ease? And in other places you might feel totally uncomfortable. The energy in the space is what we are picking up on. It's definitely a benefit to have our own homes be a place where we can relax and enjoy ourselves. The space should work for us, so that we feel that this is the best place to be, the place that we want to be more than any other: home, sweet home!

Vastu Shastra is one of the texts found in the Vedas, an ancient body of knowledge from India. Vastu explains how natural laws are universal, and that when we learn to apply these laws to our home or office, it makes our space, and our lives, more beautiful.

Vastu Shastra is India's sacred science of architecture, and it is a sister science of Ayurveda, both dating back more than 6,000 years. Vastu gives us guidelines for arranging our environments so that they are in alignment with the energy of the universe.

Buddhist monks brought Vastu from India to China, where over the years it became Feng Shui. Feng Shui literally means wind and water. It is the ancient Chinese science of placement, of working with the energies in your environment to make them conducive to your living space. With Feng Shui in place you feel more comfortable, and things come more easily to you. It helps nature to work with you, to achieve your goals, and to be your best. We probably spend more time at home that we do anywhere else, so it's important that our homes reflect ourselves and our lives in the best possible way.

◦◦ GETTING STARTED WITH FENG SHUI ◦◦

Clearing the clutter and debris in your home and in your personal life is the first step of Feng Shui and it costs you nothing. Clutter is trapped energy that has a far-reaching effect physically, mentally, emotionally and spiritually. Clutter makes you feel unorganized, confused, keeps you in the past, congests your body, and leaves you feeling lethargic and tired. And all of this can easily translate into excess weight on the body. Ridding yourself of clutter (even things which were once of value to your life) makes room in your life for what you really want and need now.

10 Tips to Clear the Clutter:

- *The 3 Questions:* Does it lift your energy? Do you use it? Do you love it? If you answer no to these questions, it's time to let it go.

- *Ready, Set, Shift that energy!* Set kitchen timer for 30 minutes and clear a small area such as a kitchen drawer. You will probably find you are feeling more energized and might have trouble stopping!

- *A Place for Everything – Put it back!* How many times have you tossed a magazine on the table, intending to get back to it? Is it still on the coffee table? There's no point in setting up an organization system if you don't use it.

- *Less is more* – The great majority of what is stored or saved is never used again - that applies to papers, clothes, magazines etc. Go paperless as much as you can – just be sure to keep your computer files organized so that it's clutter-free!

- *Finish what you've started* – Make a list of what needs to be done.

A "Honey – do" list for yourself: this could include letters or phone calls you need to make, someone you need to apologize to, or an appliance that doesn't work. Then set out to complete these things. They have all been draining your energy.

Get into good habits – Sort mail daily and file your paperwork. Have a place to put things so you don't waste time looking for them.

A full closet and nothing to wear – for some reason we hang onto clothes thinking they will come back in style or we will lose the weight we need to fit back into them. Ask yourself these questions: "Do my clothes represent who I am now?" "Do they make me feel good about myself?" If your closet is filled with clothes you no longer need, donate them to charity. Open up space in your closet for new things to come in.

Kitchen and Cupboards – Do you have any non-perishable items that you know you won't eat? Donate them to a food bank or offer them to your neighbor. Get rid of outdated food items in the refrigerator and give it a good cleaning.

Take a Trip to the Library – Not to get more books, but to donate the ones that no longer serve you. Share the knowledge you gained with someone else who may benefit from these books. Aim to have a collection of books in your home that represent you as you are today, not who you were in the past.

Shop Mindfully – the next time you go shopping, ask yourself before you buy something, "Do I really love this and need it?" "What am I willing to part with, in order to have this?" Remember that you have choices in everything you purchase. If you're on the fence about an item, make a note of it, and walk away. If you decide you still need, or want, that item in a few days and that it's in your budget, go ahead and get it. Too often our impulses get the best of us and we end up with way more stuff that we use.

Life engenders life. Energy creates energy.
It is by spending oneself that one becomes rich.
-Sarah Bernhardt

As you identify and release your clutter, you free up the energy held there for more constructive purposes. Your life may take off in ways you never thought possible.

What you want is available to you, but there may be no room in your home or your life for it as things are now. Letting go of what no longer serves you must occur before more treasures can come into your life. Releasing clutter can help you clear life patterns that are no longer of benefit to you. The simple act of clearing clutter can transform your life by releasing negative emotions, generating energy and allowing you to create space in your life for the new things you want to achieve.

Begin today by choosing one area to begin with, such as a counter top that has accumulated an entire month of junk mail. You'll get more, unfortunately – it seems to keep coming! Keep the clutter-busting simple by focusing on one area at a time. If you look at the whole picture, you might become overwhelmed and not do anything. As you eliminate the clutter from your environment, visualize what it is that you are making room for.

⌀ GREEN CLEANING ⌀

Once the clutter is gone, get cleaning! In my household I've made an effort to be green by only using natural cleaning products. I was a little skeptical at first that they could do the job as well as the "heavy duty" cleaners, but I found that these natural products not only clean just as well, they smell so much better. Remember to think of your environment as an extension of your body – and think about what you are putting onto the surfaces and into the air of your home.

I've become so sensitive to the smell of cleaning products now; it's just awful to be in a wonderful restaurant and then go into their restroom and be bombarded by toxic odors from their harsh cleansers. Look for cleaners and solvents that are biodegradable, but also made up of nontoxic, renewable ingredients that will break down quickly without negative effects to the environment and the wastewater where it goes. To make it easy, look for brands that have created just for this purpose. Ed Begley's line of cleaning products is just one example. His "Begley's Best" All-Purpose cleaner is made with citrus fruits and other natural ingredients. Best of all, 100% of proceeds go to non-profit groups.

Nothing in nature is isolated.
Nothing is without reference to something else.
Nothing achieves meaning apart from that which neighbors it.
-Goethe

You can also make your own cleaning products very easily using ingredients you probably already have on hand. Doing this saves you tons of money over buying commercial products – and you can help cut down on packaging by re-using the same spray bottles and containers over and over again.

Here's what you'll need:

- White Vinegar

- Baking Soda

- Liquid dish soap

- Tea tree oil

- Spray bottles and glass jars

Scrubbing Cleanser:
- Mix baking soda with dish soap to make a paste that is the consistency of frosting. Spread the mix onto a sponge to wash shower walls, toilets, or bathtubs. Safe for cleaning the oven and refrigerator, too.

Glass Surface Cleaner:
- Put 1 teaspoon dish soap with 6 Tablespoons of white vinegar and 4 cups of water into a spray bottle. Shake it up to mix.

Deodorizer:
- Fill up a spray bottle with mostly water and about 5 percent white vinegar. Use this to deodorize your cutting board in the kitchen. It also helps to get rid of pet smells when cleaning the litter box.

Banish Mold:
- White vinegar all by itself can kill about 80 percent of mold. Just pour it in a spray bottle and shoot the moldy area and let it dry by itself. It's a bit of a strong smell, but it goes away in a few hours. Another remedy for mold: Mix 2 teaspoons of tea tree oil with 2 cups of water in a spray bottle.

A house is no home unless it contain food
and fire for the mind as well as for the body.
-Margaret Fuller

❧ TAKING CARE OF OUR LIVING SPACE ❧

"Chi" is used in Feng Shui as the word for energy. "Prana" has a similar meaning in Vastu. Picture wind flowing through a room and circulating, that's the idea behind Chi and Prana. It's positive, it helps us to breathe, and thrive. In both Vastu and Feng Shui, our homes are regarded as sacred places; our environment is an extension of ourselves. So it is very important that we maintain our homes to keep the positive energy flowing well, just as we maintain the hygiene and health of our bodies.

It is important to fix and repair everything in your home, office and garden to maintain that good chi. Oftentimes, we hold onto items that are in need of repair, but never get around to repairing them. Broken items are symbolic of a broken life and we definitely don't want that energy around us.

How much stuff do you have that needs a screw, a dab of glue, a stitch or two? Make time to sort through these items and determine what you really want and what you know you will never fix. Determine the value of this item and if it is truly something you want to hang on to, take the time to fix it or take it to someone who will fix it for you. If you are ready to part ways with the item, then place it in the trash, sell it or donate it, but get rid of it. You won't miss is, and you'll feel so much better.

There is much symbolism used in Feng Shui and the more you learn about this art, the easier it will become for you to make these connections. These include:

- Clutter and broken items are symbolic of clutter of the mind, holding onto the past, and things which no longer work.

-Windows are considered the eyes of chi and affect your clarity, so replace broken window panes and clean the windows. If you're having a hard time "seeing" things, take a look at your windows.

-Broken or blocked doors block the voice of the adult.

-Plumbing represents our digestive system, so repair leaky faucets and clogged drains.

-Electricity and electrical devices represent our neurological system, so tend to your electrical needs - you don't want to 'short-circuit'.

-A sticking door or two doorknobs banging together, can contribute to tension between partners, so ease a tight fit. Tie red ribbons on doorknobs that bang against one another.

-Garbage cans should be put away and always covered with a lid.

-Toilets, sinks, tubs and shower stalls are drains. Connected with the water element, these are symbolic of your wealth. Keep your toilet lids down and close the drain plugs and bathroom doors to avoid draining your wealth.

Satisfaction lies in the effort,
not in the attainment.
Full effort is full victory.
-Mohandas K. Gandhi

The main entrance to your home or building is the main 'mouth' of Chi. Symbolically this is where all of the chi enters the building. It is important that the main entrance be clear, open and well defined. Below are tips to help you strengthen the entrance to your home or office:

-Eliminate obstructing clutter that blocks your path.

-Check for a squeaky door, broken handle, uneven doorframe, uneven steps or a broken doorbell.

-Check your doorknobs, repair broken hardware and add oil until the door opens flawlessly.

- Clean the entrance area and get rid of cobwebs and dirt.

- Make sure the entrance is well lit, as good lighting will create a flow of good energy into your home.

- Make sure that the access from the street or sidewalk to your home or business is clear, so that people can easily see the entrance door.

The important thing for you to remember is that all these things affect the way chí flows through your home and workplace. Although this energy is invisible, it is there. Feng Shui provides us with the tools to harness this energy and put it to work in our favor.

As chí circulates through the home, it begins to develop certain forms and invisible energy patterns. These patterns of energy form the chí that enters our bodies. The chí in our bodies in turn sends out these energy patterns like a telegraph to the world. The energy then draws to it, like a magnet, certain life situations (e.g., relationships, jobs, etc.) that reflect the same type of energy patterns that our chí is sending out.

By learning to detect how the chí flows through and around your house, you can then locate the areas where energy is blocked, stagnant, oppressive, or flowing too strongly. Bringing things back into order may be as simple as placing a plant in the corner, adding extra light to a room, or perhaps a splash of color on a wall. By learning how to work with the energy in your home, you can ultimately shape and alter the many different situations in your life.

⚬⚬ DE-STRESS YOUR WORK SPACE ⚬⚬

For many of us, our office space is our home away from home. We spend a lot of time there, so it's important to make that environment feel good to us, so that we can work most optimally and efficiently.

An office with no windows creates a LOT of stress. We need natural light, and that connection with nature. So if you're stuck in one of those offices on the inside wall of the building, you've got to work to bring nature in to you! An office with conflicting personalities also creates a lot of stress, as do deadlines, budgets and overly long meetings. What to do? Make your personal office your sanctuary!

- Chances are that plants won't thrive, so bring in silk plants for the same green, airy feeling. If there's room, make it a leafy tree! Or have fresh flowers sent to your office once a week – then you also have the benefit of a beautiful fragrance.

- Whenever possible, avoid florescent lighting, which is unnatural and stress producing. Bring in your own lamps and bulbs, preferably ones that are "full-spectrum" and more like sunlight.

- The sound of water can be both relaxing and cooling – so when tempers flare, a little desk-top fountain will help mellow you out. Another good way to bring the element of water into your office is with a little fish bowl and some fish. Even feng-shui says that they don't have to be real fish (don't stress yourself further by having to clean the tank!) – just the idea of fish is enough to make things feel calmer. You can use figurines, or pictures of fish. The goldfish represent prosperity, another added benefit!

- Decorate with colors that you love, that reflect your personality. Avoid the red/black combinations, which tend to produce more stress and anxiety – but other than that, pretty much anything goes. Just use combinations that make you feel good. Cool tones like blue are cooling and healing, earth tones are warm and grounding, yellow helps you pay attention and concentrate, orange is happy and joyful, green is balancing.

- De-clutter. Follow the OHIO rule: Only Handle It Once! Don't get buried under a pile of papers. You want to be able to find things easily – so keep files, rather than piles.

- Keep ONE calendar and write everything down. And have it with you always! Then you won't get stressed out from forgetting something important.

I believe in hard work.
It keeps the wrinkles out of the mind and the spirit.
-Helena Rubinstein

◦⊛ **THE THREE SOURCES OF POWER** ⊛◦
In our interior environments there are three sources of good energy.

⸱Fresh air, warmth and light. How we deal with these powerful
sources and thereby stimulate the flow of energy in our environment is totally up to us.

Fresh Air
Without air, we simply would not exist. Air provides us with oxygen,
which allows us to breathe. If there is too little oxygen in a room,
the air feels sticky, musty, and stale. It is our natural instinct to
open the doors and windows to obtain "fresh" air.

In every home there are two areas where smells can infiltrate the
entire home – the kitchen and the bathroom. Smokers put an abrupt
halt to fresh air and some hobby rooms, where people solder, paint,
varnish, and glue, are enveloped in acrid air.

Human scents can also weaken the air. Offices are often bogged
down by the scents of various hairsprays, gels, colognes, perfumes,
and dry cleaned clothing worn by the employees. Diseases also have
their own smells and cause the air to become heavy and stagnant.

There are numerous causes for the air losing its freshness, and
opening up windows to let new air in on a regular basis is the sim-
plest solution. However, certain rooms need extra help.

Some bathrooms contain an entire family's dirty laundry. A simple
remedy for this is to place a few drops of pure essential oil onto a
fragrance stone and place it on top of the clothes bin or on a shelf
near the clothes bin. Fragrance stones can be made from any porous
stone. Use caution with pure essential oils. Most should never be
applied directly to the skin and a few (2-4) drops are all that are
necessary. Orange, cinnamon and lavender are all good choices.

Always use the ventilation fan when cooking in the kitchen. This
draws the smells out of the area and helps to circulate the air. It's a
good idea to use a fragrance stone, aromatherapy diffuser, or pot-
pourri in the kitchen for "scent cleansing". Never leave greasy, smelly
pots and pans in the kitchen sink overnight. It is not a good way to
begin your morning, as it is symbolic of an incomplete task. If you
don't tend to it before you go to the office, it will remain in the back

of your mind throughout the day and cause you to be distracted. Additionally, take out the trash after the evening meal. Much of what we throw away has "smelly" qualities and can create a not-so-pleasant aroma the next day. Always keep a lid on garbage containers.

Warmth

Each of us has a personal temperature sensor that lets us know whether we feel comfortable or not. Many people are very uncomfortable when the temperature falls below 73°F. They shiver and reach for the nearest blanket. Others wear T-shirts, shorts and sandals at 32°F. When we heat our homes, we generally have some control over how warm we would like to have it.

Temperatures slightly cooler than in the living areas are ideal for healthy sleep, but there shouldn't be a breeze hitting you in the face when you enter the bedroom. A pleasant and cozy warmth is necessary in the living room, where you would like to relax. The activities that take place in a work room, will be the deciding factor for temperature control.

The most perfect source of heat is from a visible fire. The location of a tiled stove, or a fireplace should be as central as possible so that the warmth of the fire can radiate in all directions like a shining sun. If your fireplace is intended as a decoration, it is still important to use it on a regular basis during the cold season. A fireplace or oven that does not burn is a symbol of "extinguished" fire.

Light

Light is probably the most interesting source of good energy because we have enormous potential to optimize it. Since light plays a major role in Feng Shui, here are a few tips:

⟡ KITCHEN ⟡

There are many benefits to having good light in the kitchen. We prepare our food there and the amount of light determines how well we can see what we do. However, the quality of the light can also contribute a great deal toward how we "experience" the food and how we ultimately treat it. When working in a poorly lit kitchen, it is challenging to see the beautiful colors and quality of the food. The most vibrant colored meal will appear to be dull in poor lighting. What affect does that have on your mood? On the other hand, if the fruit, meat, or vegetables are glowing in a well-lit environment, we find them much more appealing to eat.

Working in a well-lit kitchen promotes healthy eating habits. It allows you to enjoy being in the kitchen, creates a positive eating environment, and therefore makes a valuable contribution to your health and increases your sense of well-being. In a poorly lit kitchen, the meals are unappetizing; we cook less, and then eat quickly and without much enjoyment. Who would have thought lighting could make such a difference to our health?

Even if our efforts of attention seem for years
to be producing no result, one day a light
that is in exact proportion to them will flood the room.
-Simone Weil

⤞ BATHROOM ⤝
Public restrooms are infamous for their unpleasant atmospheres. These facilities usually have a bluish-cold lighting that causes us to keep our visit as short as possible. On the other hand, the restrooms in a luxury hotel are quite comfortable and welcoming. We feel refreshed by the golden light and golden tones of the mirror there.

Gold tone mirrors may not allow us to see things as clearly, but the light flatters our skin and surrounds us with a shimmer of warmth and a touch of elegance. The choice of lighting we use in our homes can determine how much we enjoy our visit to the bathroom. Use warm lighting and gold tone mirrors to create an environment of relaxation, warmth, and elegance.

⤞ HALLWAY ⤝
In some floor plans, the hallway runs through the middle of the home or apartment and subdivides the remaining areas into different rooms. Hall lighting fixtures are usually not given much attention. However, in Feng Shui, the center of any home corresponds to health, so hall lighting should be of the utmost importance. The light in the middle of the home has the function of a sun that wants to send power into all the adjoining rooms. The more radiant the sun, the greater the energy will be. Select a hall light that is bright and reminiscent of the sun at high noon.

∘« LIVING AREAS »∘

It is important to feel sense of well-being in the living areas. The light must correspond with the needs that you have in each respective room: quality lighting for watching TV, good and bright light for reading, and warm light for snuggling. However, the light should not be blinding. If you like halogen lamps or track lighting, be sure to direct the bulbs so that no one is looking into harsh light. All lamps should be covered with shades, rather than exposing a bare bulb.

∘« DEAD CORNERS »∘

Every home has a "dead corner" somewhere. These are areas in which dust likes to collect. The energy cannot circulate freely in a corner and this area usually becomes limp. A standard lamp will work well in these areas, but using a crystal lamp is ideal. Add a few plants and a static corner can be transformed into a comfortable retreat.

∘« ACCESSORIES »∘

Most of us have a few treasures and decorative items in our homes. Quite frequently, these precious things simply gather dust and the energy around them becomes more and more weak. You can use track lighting to showcase your treasures or create a space in a bookcase for a decorative object. When you additionally illuminate the object, you are activating the energy of joy. There are special lighting fixtures that can be installed above the frames of pictures. Some rooms are completely transformed just by illuminating the pictures on the wall.

∘« HEALING GARDENS »∘

"Where is the fountain that throws
up these flowers in a ceaseless outbreak of ecstasy?"
-Rabindranath Tagore

Having your own garden is a great way to remember our connection with nature. They help us to feel at peace, and keep us grounded. All over the world, throughout history, gardens have been used to aid in the healing process. For a period of time, while 20th century medical technology flourished, the use of healing gardens had diminished. But now, with the increased interested in alternative therapies and integrative medicine, which emphasizes healing the whole person – body, mind and spirit – the idea of the garden as a healing element has been revived. Research has shows that viewing vegetation, as opposed to urban scenes, creates a state of wakeful relaxation. Here are some ideas for making your own healing garden:

- Add a water element, either a fountain or a pond.

- Make sure the garden is visually pleasing. Use soft, cool, mellow colors like pastels, violets, and white.

- Make sure the ground is even, and not too sloped, so that it is safe to walk around.

- Incorporate elements that will attract wildlife, like bird feeders and birdbaths and berry-producing shrubs.

- You may also want to include some medicinal plants in your garden, like lavender for its aromatherapy benefits, and aloe vera, which is good for sunburn.

- Create some spaces where you can sit and meditate, or just enjoy the view.

⌘ FEED THE BIRDS ⌘

We're big on birds around my house. My husband has a couple of bird feeders, and a big book where he can look up all the varieties of birds that come to visit. My step-sister, Debby Kaspari, is the bird expert in our family. She looks at birds from an artist's point of view, and paints them absolutely beautifully! I have a painting that she did for us of a Snowy Egret hanging in my entry way and I just love it. Debby gave us a terrific recipe for bird food and I thought I'd share with you:

Melt together 1 cup of lard and 1 cup of peanut butter. Stir in 2 cups of quick oats, 2 cups of yellow cornmeal and 1 cup of flour. Spread into a cookie sheet and let cool. Store in a plastic airtight container and crumble up to feed to the birds. They love it!

"A home is not a mere transient shelter:
its essence lies in its permanence, in its capacity
for accretion and solidification, in its quality of representing,
in all its details, the personalities of the people who live in it."
-H.L. Mencken

◦⊷ HOME DÉCOR BASICS ⊶◦

Sure, it would be nice to hire a decorator to swoop in and make your space all pretty and perfect. But it's a lot more fun to take on the project and create an environment that is all our own. It's so worth it to play with what you already have. Move furniture around and see where it fits both aesthetically and energetically. What looks good to you? What feels good to you? Seasonally you can change out accessories and colors to fit in with what nature has going on outside. Some basic things to think about:

- Think of a purpose for each room. A living room is for living, socializing, entertaining. Make sure you have the space set up for that. Set aside areas for conversation, with tables nearby for drinks and snacks. For maximum efficiency and comfort, a coffee table should be placed 18 inches from the couch or chair.

- Use color. A well-designed room will have one or two dominant colors and an accent color. A room with too many colors will be confusing and make you feel unsettled. A monochromatic room will feel dull and boring. It's all about balance. You can decorate with balancing colors for your dosha, or Ayurvedic mind/body type, to help you feel more comfortable. Vatas do best with warm, calming colors like green and yellow. Pittas thrive around cool colors that help to balance out their heat: silver, blue, and white are best. And Kaphas are most at home around vibrant, stimulating colors like red, gold, and orange.

Styles, like everything else, change. Style doesn't.
-Linda Ellerbee

- Use artwork. Artwork adds a lot of color and personality to a room. And it doesn't have to be expensive! You can frame a favorite poster, or create your own masterpiece with canvas and paint.

- Plants add a lot of life to the room. Live plants are great because they help to keep the air fresh. But if you're prone to killing plants, you might choose the ease of a silk plant or flower arrangement instead. When it gets dusty, simply rinse off and allow it to dry in the sun.

- Keep framed photos of friends and family. This helps to remind us of what is important in life, our relationships! A group of pictures displayed on a table makes for a great conversation piece. Choose complementary, rather than matching, frames to add visual interest.

⤎⟡ ALTARS ⟡⤏

Vastu shows us how to create altars for ourselves to attract or enhance certain energies in various areas of our lives. In India, there are altars in just about every home, temple, or building. I love the beauty and meaning behind altars, so I have placed one in my office, one in the entryway to my home, and one in my bedroom.

Altars are a beautiful and meaningful addition to any home. Altars in India originate from the Hindu tradition, and honor the divine in its many forms. This is an area where you can place items of significance to you, items that remind you of your connection with the divine. Altars can also be used to help us focus on what is important to us. They can help us to create more of what we want in our lives.

For example, a relationship altar can be used to enhance the relationship that you're in, or to draw to you the relationship you desire. An altar helps to focus our intentions.

Some tips for creating your relationship altar:

- Include representations of each of the five elements (air, space, fire, water, and earth).

- Include an offering tray, with personal and meaningful items.

- Include items in pairs: two fish, two birds, two hearts – these are all symbolic of successful relationships.

- Include items that represent love to you: photographs, flowers, hearts.

¯Activate your altar by lighting a candle or incense on the altar. Ring a bell to purify the energy in the environment and focus the mind on the present moment.

¯Spend some time each day in front of your altar meditating or simply lighting the candle and giving attention to your intention.

❖❈ **ENTERTAINING** ❈❖

It's wonderful to open our doors to family, friends and neighbors and invite them in. Having people we love around us lifts our energy, and good energy builds up in a home over time. Over the years I think we've gotten away from entertaining at home because we're so busy, and throwing a party seems like more of a chore than a pleasure. But we don't have to throw a formal affair – the idea is just to get a group together and share each other's company. It's so refreshing to sit around and just talk, face to face, instead of posting messages on each other's Facebook pages for a change!

The ornament of a house is the friends who frequent it.
There is no event greater in life than the appearance
of new persons about our hearth, except it be the progress
of the character which draws them.
-Ralph Waldo Emerson

Rather than putting pressure on yourself to do all the work – allow your guests to each bring a dish or a beverage. It doesn't have to be homemade, just something they like. You can have a theme, or go with a simple pot-luck.

The holiday season is a time when people often gather to celebrate. There are a few elements that make up any successful party. First, the atmosphere - whether your location is a home, an office or a restaurant, dress up the place to look festive, different than it looks every day.

Second, the entertainment - have something for your guests to do. It can be listening to music, playing games, creating a project together. Have some table topics handy to keep the conversation lively and break the ice with people who have just met each other.

And third, the food. As a vegan I am particularly sensitive to this! Too many times I have been to parties where there is just nothing for me to eat. Many people have dietary needs these days. One of my son's friends cannot have gluten or wheat products. A lot of my friends are lactose intolerant, and they're frustrated when they find everything drenched in dairy. It is important to have a variety of foods available so that there is something for everyone. And for beverages, do something different than just soda. Spiced cider with cinnamon sticks, cranberry juice with ginger ale, or hot chocolate with peppermint sticks are just a few examples. Cheers!

CHAPTER 5

BEAUTY
FROM THE INSIDE OUT

Beauty is eternity gazing at itself in a mirror.
- Khalil Gibran

According to Ayurveda there are three pillars of beauty. First is outer beauty. This we can see as clear skin, lustrous hair, and radiant health. Second is inner beauty. This is exemplified in a keen mind, self-confidence, and a warm, loving personality. And third is lasting beauty. This is when we look and feel younger than our chronological age.

Clear, glowing skin, and shiny hair are some of the hallmarks of beauty. Although it shows on the outside, beauty comes from within. When we are happy, we smile, and it is beautiful. We might have on designer clothes, but our best accessory is always our smile. There is a certain calm and confidence that we carry with us when we know who we are. All of this comes from following an enlightened lifestyle. Our health also plays a huge role in how beautiful we feel. Make-up only goes so far in helping to improve our appearance. When we are in optimum health our skin looks and feels good even without make-up. Some of the best beauty secrets from come from Ayurveda.

⤙ SKIN CARE ⤚

Our skin covers our body, and connects us to our environment. The skin is where we feel the sense of touch, and where we experience pain, temperature changes, and pressure.

We know that when we eat food, we need to take care to eat fresh foods, and to avoid preservatives and chemicals. The lotions and products that we apply to the skin are basically ingested by the skin in much the same way. Yes, the skin "eats" what we feed it. We need to be need careful to use natural products. The basic rule of thumb in Ayurveda is "if you can't eat it, do not put it on your skin!" So part of The Perfect Balance Diet is looking at what we are ingesting in this way, and how we are taking care of our bodies with the various products we use.

Think about it: would you eat cetyl alcohol, sodium lauryl sulfate, or red dye #17? These are very common ingredients in many popular brand-name moisturizers and soaps. We have to read the labels on our beauty products the same way we read the labels on the foods we eat. There are many synthetic and petrochemical ingredients in personal care products. Pick up any bottle of lotion, shampoo, or toothpaste in your home now and you can see which natural ingredients they contain, and how much they contain. According to the FDA's personal care products packaging standards, the further the name of an ingredient is down the list on a label, the less of that ingredient the product contains.

You'll find mineral oil in commercial lotions, creams and baby care products quite often. Mineral oil is a clear, liquid oil with no scent and it does not spoil. It is produced as a byproduct of the distillation of gasoline from crude oil. Mineral oil is leftover liquid, and because there is so much of it, it is very inexpensive. It actually costs more money to dispose of mineral oil, than to buy it.

The skin is the body's largest organ and plays an important role in maintaining overall health. However, mineral oil is foreign to the human body. Mineral oil acts as a thin layer on the skin. It is difficult to absorb and clogs the pores, which slows the skin's ability to eliminate toxins. After the oil is eventually absorbed, it is broken down by the liver and passes through the intestinal tract, where it may interfere with the absorption of fat-soluble vitamins. Mineral oil basically steals important vitamins from the body, vitamins that the body will not be able to replace. This can eventually lead to nutritional deficiencies. The medical community has said that mineral oil should never be taken orally or used as an ingredient in medications. So, remember the rule: "If you can't eat it, do not put it on your skin!" Fortunately, we have many alternatives to mineral oil.

Skin is alive, and to best give life back to the skin, we need to use natural products. Plant-based products, meaning flowers, vegetables, fruits, and herbs are nourishing and beneficial to the skin. Vegetable oils are extracts from plants. The best oils are organic, which means that the plants they are made from have not been subject to any chemical sprayed or fertilized. There are many beauty products that are made with these natural ingredients and you can often find them in health food stores. I recommend a wonderful line of beauty products from Maharishi Ayurveda® called "Youthful Skin" that you can find on my website: DoshaSmart.com. There is a cleanser, toner, moisturizer, eye serum, body lotion and more.

Ayurda® is another company that makes a wonderful range of Ayurvedic beauty products. What makes their line unique is that it is dosha specific, so you can really customize your skin care routine to the dosha of your skin. You can find their entire line at DharmaSmart.com.

Vata skin tends to be dry and rough. Because it is thinner than other skin, it may show its age more quickly. Vata skin is cool to the touch. When you shake hands with a Vata person you notice this right away! Vata skin gets dehydrated easily, so it needs lots of moisture to stay in balance.

Abhyanga, a warm oil self-massage is great for all the doshas, and it is especially beneficial for Vata types. It helps to keep the skin lubricated, and it helps the skin to release toxins. Abhyanga also helps to tone the muscles and soothe the nervous system. The massage can be done in the morning before your shower, or in the evening before bed. Start by warming the oil to skin temperature, and drizzle a small amount of oil into the palms of your hands. Massage the top of your scalp (on days when you wash your hair), pay particular attention to the circumference of your ears, and the soles of your feet. Massage with long strokes on your limbs, and round strokes on your joints. It's best to leave the oil on the body for 20 minutes before washing it off in a warm shower or bath.

Pitta skin is sensitive. People with pitta skin often have fair skin and freckles. Pitta is made up of fire and water, so as you can imagine, there is a lot of heat in this dosha. Pittas run warm, and when you hold their hands, you will feel it! They are prone to redness, rashes, and rosacea. To balance the heat, Pittas need cooling treatments for their skin. Rose water is cooling and soothing to Pitta skin. Keep a spray handy to use whenever you feel the heat rising. Definitely stay out of the sun when you can, and use sun protection on your skin at all times.

Summertime is Pitta season, and this is a time when we all need to be a little more mindful about our skin care in the sun. Ayurveda has these tips for us:

- Avoid exposure to the sun when angry, hungry or upset. These factors increase Pitta, which makes the skin more susceptible to sun damage.

- Protect yourself with sunscreen, and also with clothing, hats, long sleeves, and sunglasses during times when you are most sensitive.

- Avoid the mid-day sun. Early morning sun is more gentle to the skin.

- Cool yourself from the inside by eating cool foods, salads, fresh sweet pears, and raisins. Avoid hot foods, like peppers and chilies.

- Cool down skin with a mask made of watermelon puree. Avoid the eye area, and rinse off with lukewarm water after about 15 minutes.

Kapha skin is thick and soft, and tends to be oily. Because Kapha skin is naturally moist, it tends to age more slowly. Kaphas can have large pores, especially in the T-Zone of the face. Kaphas need to exfoliate to help the skin release built-up ama, or toxins. An herbalized clay mask is ideal for this!

⊶ ACNE ⊷
Acne is a common skin disease that affects more than 85% of the population at some point in their lives. Acne is more common in men than women during adolescence, and more common in women than men during adulthood. Ayurveda says that acne is an imbalance of all three doshas: Vata, Pitta and Kapha, with the main

cause being the aggravation of the Pitta dosha. Pitta is made up of a combination of fire and water, hence the heat, or redness, of the skin. Since a Pitta imbalance is deep in the physiology, creams and topical treatments just mask the symptoms of acne. Ayurveda recommends a Pitta diet and lifestyle routine to tackle the disease at the root cause. Meditation and yoga help to ease stress, which is a contributing factor. When experiencing a breakout of acne, try making a paste of turmeric powder and water and applying to the blemishes with a cotton ball. Turmeric is an antibiotic and antibacterial so will help calm the eruptions.

✧❈ THE MIRACLE PLANT ❈✧

Aloe Vera is often referred to as a "miracle plant" in Ayurveda, and it is an ingredient in many ayurvedic beauty products. The Aloe Vera plant is a succulent, and its leaves contain a liquid that is made up of 96% water and the rest is a combination of amazing healing ingredients like Vitamins A, B, C, E, calcium, amino acids and enzymes. The gel from the Aloe Vera plant can be applied to the skin to help heal cuts, insect bites, bruises, and skin conditions such as eczema and poison ivy.

Aloe Vera has both antibacterial and antifungal properties. It can help the skin manufacture collagen, and it is absorbed into the skin four times faster than water making it extremely moisturizing.

✧❈ VEGETABLE OILS ❈✧

There are many different varieties of vegetable oils, and Ayurveda recommends a few different ones for each skin type.

- If you have dry, or Vata skin, look for Sesame, Avocado, Olive, Almond, or Walnut Oil.

- If you have sensitive, or Pitta skin, use Almond, Coconut, Sunflower, Apricot Kernel or Olive Oil.

- If you have oily, or Kapha skin, the best oils for you are Canola, Corn, Safflower, Mustard, Grapeseed, Apricot Kernel or Almond Oil.

You can use vegetable oils as a natural moisturizer, or for massage. You can slather on the oil before your shower to give your skin an extra treat! Vegetable oils are so good you'll want to keep them near every sink in your home, to moisturize your hands a little bit after you wash them. This keeps your hands feeling soft and looking young. DoshaSmart.com has a wide variety of oils, including specially herbalized oils based on ancient Indian recipes.

The Sanskrit word for oil is "snigdha." Sanskrit has many layers of meaning, and translated, snigdha means oil, fat and also, love! Oil creates smoothness, lubrication, and vigor. It is nourishing, like love. When we use oil in a massage, we are taking care of ourselves, and coating ourselves with love. The opposite of oily is dry, or "ruksha." Dryness creates dehydration. Dry weather aggravates vata, and causes dry skin. Fear, nervousness, anxiety and loneliness are also dry. Love is the antidote! So to balance ruksha, coat the skin with oil, or love. Then take a warm shower after the application of oil, and the skin, kidneys and colon are also nourished.

☞☜ COCONUT OIL ☞☜

Coconut oil is popular in Ayurveda as a massage oil to balance pitta, and as a conditioner for hair. I've come across some other uses for coconut oil that might surprise you – but how wonderful to be creative, and health conscious at the same time!

- While coconut oil is conditioning to the hair, it also can help cure dandruff. Just massage a little bit onto the scalp. This is a very gentle treatment that can even be used on children and babies.

- There are strong antifungal agents in coconut oil, so it can be used to treat athlete's foot, ringworm, thrush and yeast infections.

- The moisturizing properties of coconut oil make it good for helping many skin conditions like eczema. It can also be used as a make-up remover, or as a lip balm.

- Because coconut oil also has antimicrobial and anti-inflammatory properties, it can be used as a cream for small cuts and scrapes, protecting against infection while helping the skin to heal.

- Mixed with baking soda, coconut oil can be used as a natural toothpaste.

❧❦ STRESS ❦❧

According to Ayurveda, stress can trigger, or aggravate skin disorders such as acne, hives, eczema, psoriasis, rosacea, warts, cold sores and blisters. This is because skin is an organ, connected to our physiology and also our mind. Skin is affected by stress much as any other organ would be. In stressful situations the fight-or-flight mechanism kicks in, sending the flow of blood and nutrients to areas of the body that are necessary to respond to the stress, and away from areas considered non-essential, such as the skin. If this happens often enough, the skin is deprived of both blood and oxygen, making it dull, dry, and more prone to clogged pores. Stress impacts our immune system, and also our digestion. Poor digestion affects skin health because the nutrients of the foods are not properly absorbed, and the undigested impurities accumulate in the body faster than the body can get eliminate them. What to do? Ayurveda recommends a holistic system for stress management and skin health:

- Meditate to help keep the mind and emotions balanced.

- Eat a balanced diet of fresh foods recommended for your dosha.

- Avoid caffeine.

If you want to try making some great beauty treatments at home, stock up on these items at the grocery store:

- Almond Meal – mix with dry milk and sugar to cleanse dry skin, or dry milk and ground orange peel for sensitive skin. Make a paste with warm water and gently massage into the skin. Rinse with warm water and pat dry.

- Barley Meal – Mix with dry milk and ground lemon peel to cleanse oily skin. Use as above.

- Milk – if your skin is very dry, heat some milk to skin temperature and froth it, then apply as a mask to your skin.

- Bananas or avocados make great exfoliating masks for dry skin.

- Pineapple is very good for sensitive skin.

- Strawberries work really well for oily skin. The little seeds in the strawberries are like nature's perfect exfoliator!

Love is a great beautifier.
–Louisa May Alcott

◦⸙ HAIR CARE ⸙◦

According to Ayurveda both our hair and our nails are a by-product of our bones. So in order to have healthy hair, we need to maintain proper nutrition for healthy bones. If calcium and magnesium are not completely absorbed by our bones, we'll see it in our hair as split ends, hair that breaks easily, or even hair that falls out. Dairy products are a good source of calcium and magnesium, but many of us are either vegan or lactose intolerant. Luckily there are many non-dairy foods we can eat as alternatives: daikon, coconut, cooked apples, and cabbage. Sesame seeds are packed with calcium and magnesium, so sprinkle some on your breakfast cereal, on your toast, or in your salad at dinner. Sesame seeds are potent little nutritious gems; they're also a good source of copper, manganese, and iron. A gentle scalp massage with sesame oil is also beneficial because it improves circulation at the root of the hair.

Ayurveda is really big on scalp massage as a way to improve circulation and stimulate hair growth. We lose about 50-100 strands of hair a day, so we need to keep a constant supply coming! It is a good idea to treat yourself to a scalp massage once a week. If you have dry hair or dandruff, you may want to do this twice a week. If you have oily skin or hair, you can do the massage without the oil. First thing in the morning, or last thing before bed is the best time for this treatment. Start by warming 1 teaspoon of sesame oil, or your favorite oil for your dosha. Massage this into the scalp for ten minutes. Use the pads of your fingers, not your nails. Massage in a circular motion. Then wrap your head in a hot towel and leave on for about 10 minutes more. This helps replace some of the lost moisture in your hair – best conditioning treatment ever! Wash hair with a gentle shampoo. Massage increases circulation to the scalp and promotes healthy hair growth. And it feels great!

To protect the hair from sun damage, throw on a hat, especially in the summer. Don't use metal brushes or combs on your hair, they're too damaging. Instead look for natural bristle brushes and wood combs when possible.

Put a little dab of olive oil on eyelashes and eyebrows before bed and they'll get thicker over time.

Beauty is how you feel inside,
and it reflects in your eyes.
It is not something physical.
– Sophia Loren

⌐« BATH TIME! »⌐

Sure, taking a bath is a nice way to get cleaned up. But in Ayurveda a bath is so much more than that. A bath can actually be therapy! It relaxes the muscles, opens up the pores, and restores moisture to the body tissues. A bath can also clear the mind and balance emotions. Sounds wonderful, doesn't it? It's easy to prepare a healing bath, and here are a few guidelines:

- Use cleansers that are moisturizing. The idea is to help the skin absorb the water and rehydrate. The skin's moisture balance is essential for the overall health of the skin.

- Make sure the bath water is pure. Use a water filter if necessary. The water should be comfortably warm, not too hot or too cold.

- Take your time in the bath, relax and breathe deeply.

- Set the mood in the room with natural aromatherapy and soft lighting.

- Moisturize your skin after the bath.

Baths are a fantastic way to let go of the stress of the day. You can make a ritual out of your bath time with candles and soft music and some simple, natural ingredients added to your bath water. Dry milk powder is lovely for dry or sensitive skin. For dry skin, try adding a few drops of honey. And for oily skin, add a few drops of lemon oil. If you happen to have eczema or psoriasis, add licorice tea to the bath water, it is very soothing.

If you don't have time for a full bath, one option is to just soak your feet. Adding a few drops of witch hazel and lavender oil is super refreshing. If you have callouses, add some lemon juice to the water.

⌐« FOOT CARE »⌐

Bathing the feet can also help to refresh the body. There are a variety of foot soaks to help relieve and invigorate the feet. Use a small tub or a bowl large enough to that you can fill it with water to cover up to the ankles.

- For Sweaty Feet: fill the bowl with warm water, and add 6 drops each of lavender, sage, juniper and cypress essential oils. To help deodorize, add some rock salt and bay leaf to the mix.

- For Tired Feet: use the essential oils of juniper, rosemary, and lavender in your foot bath.

- To Calm and Cool the system: use the essential oil of sandalwood in your cool water foot bath.

- For a Head Cold: add ginger (either fresh grated or ginger essential oil) or mustard powder to a hot foot bath. Leave your feet in until they turn red, then put on warm socks. This warms the whole body and helps to drain mucus and congestion from the head.

- For a Restful Sleep: Massage the feet with warm sesame oil or ghee. Then soak the feet in a hot herbal foot bath with warming spices such as ginger.

After your footbath, massage the feet with your favorite vegetable oil and then wear socks to bed. A foot massage is truly lovely and quite beneficial for the whole body. You'll get a great night's sleep and wake up with happy little tootsies in the morning!

Ayurvedic massage typically uses warm sesame oil, or a blend of oils and herbs specifically to balance your particular dosha. A foot massage can be a self-massage, or you can indulge your partner. The Ayurvedic massage technique doesn't involve deep muscle massage, rather the goal is to stimulate the subtle energies of the marma points and nadis (similar to acupressure points) in the body. Start with the right foot, then repeat the same steps on the left.

Here's what you do:

- Start with the point located in the middle of the arch of the foot. Massage this area with your thumb, it is good for the heart.

- Using the thumb, massage the point located in the middle of the underside of the big toe. This area regulates hormonal activity.

- Starting with the big toe, massage the underside of the base of each toe. Then massage each toe all around by gently pulling upward from the base to the top. Each toe corresponds to a major organ: brain, lungs, intestines, kidney, heart.

- Now work on the top of the foot. Using both thumbs, massage the groove between the base of the big toe and the second toe. Massage up toward the ankle until you feel the bone.

- Now hold the foot with both hands and massage upward from the toes to the ankle.

Other tips for happy feet:

- Avoid wearing shoes that are too tight, or heels that are too high.

- Keep a tennis ball under your desk at work. Kick off your shoes and roll the ball with your feet for a mini-foot massage.

- Walk around barefoot whenever you can, particularly on soft grass or sand. Ayurveda says that it is good for us to give our feet as much air as possible. Shoes trap energy around the feet and can make you feel more tired. It is also believed that shoes collect negativity, which is why they are never worn in Indian temples. Feel free to walk around your house barefoot.

Beauty, to me, is about being comfortable in your own skin.
That, or a kick-ass red lipstick.
~Gwyneth Paltrow

⊶⋙ HAND THERAPY ⋙⊷

Sometimes the hands give away our age more than the face does. We need to pay attention to our hands, that do so much work for us every day. Mudras are kind of like yoga for the hands. Mudras are hand positions, or exercises, used to balance various energies in the body. In Ayurveda, there are five elements, and each corresponds with one of the fingers. The thumb represents fire. The second finger represents air. The third finger represents space. The fourth finger, or ring finger, represents earth, and the little finger represents water. Mudras can have positive effects on our physiology. And we can get some of the same benefits by working with our hands, playing an instrument, washing our hands, and massaging our hands.

The next time you wash your hands, try consciously massaging them at the same time. Spend time on each finger, and then rub both palms together vigorously. While you're sitting at your desk, use the thumb and index finger to gently massage the "web" between each of your fingers. Place one hand on your desk, and use the second, third, and fourth fingers of the other hand to gently massage between the long bones on the back of the hand.

According to Ayurveda, the condition of our nails is a reflection of the condition of the condition of our body tissues. If we're having problems with our nails, then we need to look at the balance and nourishment of the whole body. Here are some examples of what we can find by looking at our nails:

- Horizontal indentations indicate a weakened digestion.

- Vertical ridges indicate that we are not metabolizing minerals or proteins well, and that we have a deficiency in Vitamin B12 and Iron.

- White spots indicate a calcium or zinc deficiency.

- Hang nails indicate a lack of protein, Vitamin C, and folic acid.

- Brittle nails indicate low iron or low Vitamin A, an imbalanced thyroid or kidney function and poor circulation.

- Yellowish nails indicate a liver imbalance.

- Bluish nails indicate a lung and heart imbalance.

- Pale nails indicate anemia, and low liver and kidney energy.

In addition, we can look at the particular finger where a nail has a problem, and note that there may be an imbalance in the corresponding organ.

- Thumb: *brain*

- Index finger: *lungs and colon*

- Middle finger: *small intestine*

- Ring finger: *kidney*

- Little finger: *heart and female reproductive organs*

⟿ MASSAGE AND SPA TREATMENTS ⟿

Massage is fantastic for your skin, your muscles and general relaxation. There are special massage techniques that come from various cultures around the world. More and more spas are beginning to offer Ayurvedic treatments on their menus. Here's a break-down of the options, so you know what you can order if you're lucky enough to indulge in one of these treatments:

- **Abhyanga** can be done as either a massage or a self-massage. The oil, usually infused with herbs especially chosen to help balance your dosha, penetrates the skin, relaxes the mind and body, and helps to stimulate circulation. See Chapter 8 for detailed instructions how to perform Abhyanga as a part of your daily routine.

- **Garshana** is a dry massage. Silk gloves are used to brush the skin and enhance circulation. Garshana is popular for its ability to break down cellulite over time. This massage also cleans the skin so that oil and herbs can more deeply penetrate the skin. If you want to try this treatment at home you can find Garshana gloves at DoshaSmart.com.

- **Shirodhara** comes from the Sanskrit word "Shiro" meaning head, and "Dhara" meaning flow. In this technique, flowing liquid is gently poured over the forehead. Typically a person lies down, and a metal pot is hung over the person's head. From this pot warm oil or liquid streams onto the forehead. Shirodhara is also known as the Third Eye Treatment because the third eye is located in the forehead, just above and between the eyebrows over which the liquid is poured. There is another container below the head to catch all the liquid as it flows off the body.

Oil is the most common liquid that is used in the Shirodhara treatment, and other liquids that are often used are herbalized oils, milk buttermilk, coconut water, or plain water.

Shirodhara is incredibly relaxing – it can send a person into a deep state of meditation. Shirodhara also helps to remove toxins, or "ama" from the body, and it helps to calm the mind, stabilize the nervous system and bring about positive emotions. The technique also helps nutrients within the body to flow freely to the brain, encouraging healing from within. Shirodhara has been known to help with problems such as insomnia, headache, and lack of focused attention.

In the past, we've needed to locate a spa that has the proper equipment to perform this very specialized type of treatment. But now, I've found a really wonderful, self-contained Shirodhara machine that lets you do your own Shirodhara right at home, whenever you want! You can use any of your favorite oils for the most benefit, or, you can use water and keep it really simple. Shirodhara treatments in a spa cost around $100, so if you want to have these treatments on a regular basis, with the convenience of having them in your own home, it really makes sense to get your own machine. My hubby got me one for my birthday and I absolutely love it! You can find it at DharmaSmart.com.

- **Swedana** is like a steam bath. A tent is used so the head is kept cool while the body is heated to remove toxins that have built up in the body, mind, and emotions deep within the cells. Sweating also stimulates the digestive fire, and relieves coldness, stiffness, and heaviness due to bloating. Always finish off swedana with cleansing and moisturizing the skin.

- **Udvartana** is a massage that uses an herbal paste to help the lymphatic system drain. This is an exfoliating treatment that also beautifully conditions the skin.

- **Vishesh** is a deep muscular massage. It helps open up the channel of communication to the deep tissues and improve circulation to the muscles.

- **Marma** Therapy is a technique used in Ayurvedic practice which helps to move prana through the body to assist in balancing, and healing. Prana is the Sanskrit word for energy, or life force, or breath. Marma therapy is similar to acupressure in that there are special points to which pressure is applied. There are 107 primary marma points that correspond to places on the skin. However, these points are not fixed, but can differ in location from one person to another. A sensitive therapist can locate the area of congestion and work to get the prana moving. Marma therapy can also be practiced routinely in self-care and it is a simple and effective healing technique.

Beauty is not in the face;
beauty is a light in the heart.
- Kahlil Gibran

⤸ ORAL HEALTH ⤹

The health of our mouths is an important factor to our overall physical health. In Ayurveda, brushing and flossing the teeth twice a day is an essential part of the daily routine. Tongue scraping is also recommended. Tongue scrapers, or cleaners, are typically made out of stainless steel. It takes only a moment to clean the tongue with this tool, and it helps to remove decay causing bacteria as well as encourage the removal of toxins from the digestive tract. The Sanskrit word for these toxins is "ama" and research shows that tongue cleaning is the best way remove bacteria that cause bad breath. It also helps to remove the coating on the tongue, leaving us with improved taste, and slowing the growth of plaque.

And here's more reason to be ever mindful of our oral health: Research suggests that we may be able to reduce our chance of getting heart disease by practicing good oral hygiene. There is definitely a relationship between heart health and tooth brushing. Simply by brushing your teeth you are helping yourself to have a healthier heart. British researchers have found that people who do not brush their teeth twice a day have as much as a 70% extra risk of heart disease. The main factors for heart disease are smoking and a poor diet. But after that, regular tooth brushing (at least twice a day) is also a factor, and a simple measure to take to help maintain a healthy heart. Twice daily brushing also reduces the risk of gum or periodontal disease, an infection of the tissues surrounding and supporting the teeth. Researchers recommend good oral hygiene by seeing a dentist every six months, and using products like tongue scrapers, mouthwash, and water picks.

According to Ayurveda, because the mouth is governed by the kapha dosha, bad breath, or halitosis, is a kapha disorder. However, because digestion is governed by the pitta dosha, pitta is also indirectly responsible. When the digestive fire, or agni, is not functioning properly, our digestion is off, which could lead to bad breath. Bad breath is caused when bacteria in the mouth decomposes the residue of food and releases sulfur. The sulfur is what smells bad.

Clove is commonly used in ayurvedic dental treatments. Because of its pungent taste, clove is great for balancing kapha, which helps to fight bad breath. Tulsi, or Holy Basil, can also be used to treat bad breath. Just chew a few fresh leaves right off the plant. To prevent bad breath, flavor foods with cardamom and clove. Drink lots of water throughout the day. If you can't brush and floss after every meal, at least brush twice a day, and gargle after eating.

Neem oil is one of the favorite medicinal oils used in Ayurveda, and you'll often see it as an ingredient in ayurvedic toothpaste, as it is very healing to the gums. Neem is unique in that it is antiviral, antibacterial, and also antimicrobial. The Neem tree is sometimes called the "toothbrush tree" because neem has many dental applications. In India, people often pull a twig off the tree and chew the end to form bristles, making a natural toothbrush.

As you can see, from the top of our heads to the tips of our toes, there are many wonderful ways we can take care of ourselves so that our natural beauty can shine through!

Taking joy in living is a woman's best cosmetic.
- Rosalind Russell

CHAPTER 6

UNPLUGGED
TUNING IN

If you were to ask me what was the most important experience
of my life, I would say it was learning to meditate.
For me that is the most important thing a person can do
to restore harmony and evolve to a higher state of consciousness.
-Deepak Chopra

Besides being an author, I am also a meditation instructor with The Chopra Center. Most busy people think they don't have time to meditate, but I tell them that they don't have time not to. This is where you clear your mind! And what is meditation? It is simply doing NOTHING! Sitting in silence, eyes closed... just breathe. Of course we can't stop our brains from thinking – we are thinking all the time. But we can settle those thoughts down, allow them to float by, so that we have a little peace in the mix.

Why meditate? There's a story that the Buddha was once asked "What have you gained from meditation?" Without pause, he replied "Nothing!" And then he said, "Let me tell you what I have lost: anger, anxiety, depression, insecurity, and the fear of old age and death." Meditation is as essential to the mind as nutrition is to the body. It's an important part of the Perfect Balance Diet.

⇌ CLEAR YOUR MIND WITH MEDITATION ⇌
This is how it works: Imagine your mind as a cupboard. There are all kinds of things stashed away in there – things to do, places

to go, stuff to buy, errands to run, birthdays to remember... not to mention all the "stored" items like phone numbers, multiplication tables, social security numbers, e-mail addresses and security codes. What happens is that as we're in a hurry, as we usually are, all these tidbits get crammed into the cupboard any which way. So when we want to retrieve something, the more stuff that is in there, the harder it is to find. But... we can clear our minds, give ourselves space to move things around, just as we can clear our cupboards, and keep everything all neat and orderly!

Meditation quiets our minds and allows our bodies to gain the deep rest necessary to relieve stress and fatigue. In meditation we re-connect with our true selves. This connection extends into our daily lives and results in improved health, better relationships, a renewed enthusiasm, increased creativity... and yes, more efficiency! Because we are more efficient, and spend less time worrying and stressing out, we have more time to be productive.

There are many health benefits to meditation. Doctors are increasingly citing stress as a major factor in illnesses such as depression, anxiety, high blood pressure, colds, and asthma. Much work time is lost from these health problems. Research has shown that meditation contributes to reducing stress, which has important benefits and also allows the mind and body to function optimally. Our memories are better when our minds are clear.

Just 20 -30 minutes spent in silence twice a day will add hours onto your day, and probably years onto your life.

❧ VISUAL MEDITATIONS ❧

There are many different types of meditation. An easy way to start your exploration of this practice is with visual meditations. Sit quietly and rest your eyes on an object or an image. Take this image in, and whenever thoughts come into your head to distract you away from this, go back to just looking at the image, without any agenda. Here are three common objects that are used for visual meditations:

⊶⊛ THE SHRI YANTRA ⊛⊷

A yantra is a geometric figure from the Vedic tradition. It is a visual expression of a mantra, or sacred sound. The Shri Yantra represents the mantra "OM" which loosely translated means All, or the Universal. This Yantra is composed of many triangles, some of which pass through each other to form new triangles. The triangles which point upward represent masculine energy, or Shiva. The downward pointing triangles represent feminine energy, or Shakti. Creation comes from the combination of male and female energy. This energy has unlimited potential, which is why the circles are framed by the square pointing outward on each side, to represent infinity.

By meditating on the Shri Yantra we can create peace, harmony and wealth in our lives. Wealth in the Vedic culture is defined not just as material prosperity, but as spiritual fulfillment as well.

Om shanti shanti shanti. Peace, peace, peace.

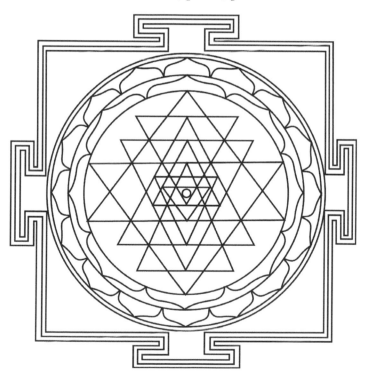

◦❖ **THE LABYRINTH** ❖◦

Labyrinths have appeared in many cultures throughout time. They are in ancient Greek floor mosaics, Scandinavian gardens, and medieval cathedrals. Because of the similarity of these various structures, they have been regarded as significant religious symbols. The labyrinth, which takes up just a small space, indicates a long and arduous path.

The ritual of walking the labyrinth reminds us to stay on the path. Sometimes we seem to be far away from our center, and other times we are led right to it. Sometimes the road is full of twists and turns, and other times the way is smooth and clear.

Meditating on the labyrinth helps to keep us centered. It helps us to remember that the answers are within. And that if we just stay on the path, wisdom will come to us.

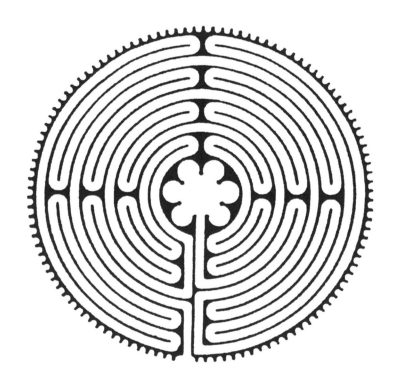

⌁⊷ **THE BUTTERFLY** ⊷⌁

The Greek word for butterfly is "psyche," which also means "soul." The butterfly undergoes a transformation. It evolves from a caterpillar to a cocoon, and then ultimately into its full glory as a beautiful winged creature. This process is a metaphor for the change that can happen to each one of us. As we learn and grow, we begin to recognize ourselves as the wonderful beings that we truly are.

Meditating on the butterfly reminds us that each day, and each moment, is a new beginning. Instead of crawling on the ground, we are free to rise above our problems, and see things from a higher perspective.

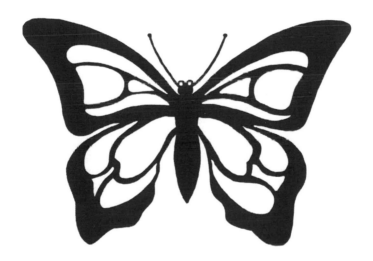

⌁⊷ **MEDITATION TECHNIQUES** ⊷⌁

Because people have many different temperaments, many different meditative techniques have been developed. If you have never meditated, you might wish to try several of the following techniques to discover which one is the best for you. If you respond to music, you can try an instrumental meditation track. If you are a visual learner, you might start with Tratak. In any case, get into the habit of meditating by setting aside quiet time each day.

Meditation is a time to let go of your daily tensions and anxieties, a time to let your mind and body relax and just be. It is also a time to gain insights into your inner resources.

✦ WITNESSING ✦

Witnessing is the purest form of meditation. It is simply sitting in meditation and watching the thoughts that come and go without judging or commenting. It is interesting to see what our moment-to-moment thoughts consist of from a completely neutral position.

✦ VIPASSANA ✦

Vipassana is a Buddhist meditation that focuses on the rise and fall of the breath. Vipassana means "breath." While the mind is engaged in focusing on your breathing it cannot focus on its usual distractions. In this meditation, your breathing should be gentle and regular. Just allow it to be the place where your mind is focused and enjoy the feeling of witnessing breathing rather than concentrating on it.

✦ ZAZEN ✦

Zazen means "just sitting." It is the basic meditation of Zen Buddhists, for whom the path of enlightenment is everyday life, lived with awareness and totality. Like all meditations, Zazen is a tool to help us rediscover the immediacy and freshness of ordinary life, as we did as children. In Zazen, you just sit and allow whatever happens to happen. Your mind will try to distract you with past and present concerns to take you away from fully experiencing the moment Zen Buddhists believe these transient thoughts are "paper tigers" and that paying attention to them only gives them more energy. In Zazen, you gain a feeling of sitting and experiencing the fact that you are not the mind and can ignore its chatter at will. If your mind is particularly rebellions, you can give it a distraction to play with, such as concentrating on the breath.

✦ TRATAK (GAZING) ✦

Another device to still the mind so that you can experience directly is Tratak, or "gazing." The object that you look at is not really important. Traditional objects include a lighted candle, a flower, a religious image, or a picture of a guru. The main point of the exercise is to keep your eyes on a central spot because not moving the eyes restricts the input of information for your brain to process. The idea is to keep your mind quiet by keeping your thoughts simple. When you start to think about something else, keep bringing your attention back to the object of your contemplation. The goal of your meditation is to feel the quality of the object, to relax, and to enjoy what you are seeing.

◦◦ LISTENING ◦◦

Meditation is centered in the idea of relaxing and non-doing. When you are thinking, you may hear but you cannot truly listen. As you center your awareness in music, chanting, or natural sounds, you experience the essence of the sound, giving yourself the experience of emptiness, clarity, and receptivity.

◦◦ MANTRA ◦◦

In mantra meditation, you produce the sounds out loud or to yourself; either way, the sounds will produce an internal effect. In the Sanskrit language, man is translated as "mind" and tra means "protection." The repetition of the mantra or sound evokes a deep and peaceful reaction throughout your body.

Mantras are energies that are thought to have always existed in the universe. They pass in succession from teacher to disciple in an unbroken chain. The mantra leads the way to meditation and to a state of nonduality. Two typical Eastern mantras are "Om" (I am) and "So-Ham" (I am That).

A mantra can be anything that you enjoy repeating. The words "peace" or "one" are often used, as are names of saints or great teachers. For example, "Om Namah Shivaya" is a Sanskrit mantra that means "the God within." It should be repeated slowly, sounding each syllable: Om/Na/Mah/Shi/Va/Ya. Another, and perhaps the most widely used mantra in the world today, is "Om Mani Padme Hum." In Sanskrit Om represents the universal energy or life-force, Mani means "jewel" or "crystal." Padme means "lotus," and Hum means "heart." "Shalom" is a Hebrew word meaning peace, often chanted in prayers. "Shalom" contains the same "ah" and "om" syllables used in other mantras.

Ram Dass, in The Only Dance There Is, explains this mantra as meaning: "The entire universe is like a pure jewel or crystal within the heat of the lotus flower, which represents myself, and it is manifest in my own heart."

Choose a mantra that feels right to you. You can chant it out loud or repeat it silently to yourself. Mantras are often used in conjunction with the Vipassana to bring about a deeper meditation.

I practice a mantra-based meditation technique that was developed by Deepak Chopra. It is called Primordial Sound Meditation. The mantra given to each individual when they learn this meditation is personal, determined by the person's birth date, time and place. If you are interested in learning this type of meditation, you can find a certified instructor in your area by visiting Chopra.com.

❧ MEDITATION IN ACTION ❧

Everything can become a meditation, including the most ordinary everyday chores. What transforms daily activities into meditation action is awareness and wholeheartedness. The application of the Zen exhortation to give undivided attention to and really feel the quality of each of your actions is exemplified in the Japanese tea ceremony and the art of flower arranging. Being present in the moment imparts an unmistakable peace, effortlessness, and enjoyment to the "little things" that make up the greater whole of life. I like to do a little "chocolate" meditation in the evening. To do this, take a small piece of dark chocolate, and put it in your mouth. Close your eyes. Sit in silence so that your sense of taste is heightened. Feel the texture of the chocolate on your tongue. Allow the chocolate to melt with your body heat. Savor the sweetness. Be fully present with the sensations that arise. Enjoy every blissful moment!

Make the most of yourself,
for that is all there is of you.
~Ralph Waldo Emerson

⌇ CHAKRAS ⌇

Chakra is Sanskrit for "wheel" or "ring." There are seven chakras, or energy centers, located along our spine. The chakras absorb vibrations from within the body and from our environment and they radiate that energy throughout our body. It is important to keep our chakras balanced, as we are healthier and happier when they can function optimally. Meditation is a great way of balancing the chakras.

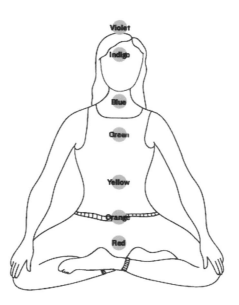

7. **The Crown Chakra or "Sahasrara"**
    - Located at the crown of the head. Opens up our spiritual connection.
    - Color: violet
    - Mantra: OM (ohm)
    - The keyword is INSPIRATION. The crown chakra influences spirituality.
    - We are more than our bodies, and through this chakra we most often feel our connection with the Universe.

6.   *The Third Eye Chakra or "Ajna"*

- Located in the middle of the brow, between and slightly above the eyebrows. Opens up our wisdom.

- Color: Indigo

- Mantra: Ksham (kshahm)

- Your keyword here is INTUITION. The third eye chakra allows us to see what we cannot see with our eyes alone. This chakra influences the brain.

5.   *The Throat Chakra or "Vishuddha"*

- Located in the center of the throat. Opens up our communication and self-expression.

- Color: Blue

- Mantra: Hum (hoom)

- The keyword for the throat chakra is EXPRESSION. This chakra influences thyroid function, and also speech. Blue brings clarity and truth to our words.

4.   *The Heart Chakra or "Anahata"*

- Located at the heart center. Opens us up to love and relationships.

- Color: Green

- Mantra: Yam (yahm)

- The keyword for the heart chakra is BALANCE. The heart chakra is in the middle, at the center of the body. Even the color green is a balance, a blend of the cool color blue and the warm color yellow. It influences circulation, respiration, and the immune system.

3.   *The Solar Plexus Chakra or "Manipura"*

- Located in the middle of the solar plexus. Opens us up to our will power and motivation.

- Color: Yellow

- Mantra: Ram (rahm)

- The keyword for the solar plexus chakra is WHOLENESS. This chakra influences the energy of digestion and absorption. The solar plexus chakra is where we feel our "gut" instincts, and it is often where we process information

2. **The Creative Chakra or "Swadhisthana"**

- Located near our reproductive organs, about two inches below the navel. Opens up our creativity and happiness.
- Color: Orange
- Mantra: Vam (vahm)
- Your keyword is STABILITY. The sacral chakra, also known as the creative chakra, influences sexual energy, as well as the energies of fertility and creativity

1. **The Base Chakra or "Muladhara"**

- Located at the base of the spine. Opens us up to being grounded.
- Color: Red
- Mantra: Lam (lahm)
- Your keyword here is POTENCY. The base chakra influences the energy of elimination. It also helps to keep you grounded.

⚬⚫ CHAKRA MEDITATION ⚫⚬

In a seated position, with your spine straight, close your eyes and relax. Take a few deep cleansing breaths.

Start with the first chakra at the base of your spine. Breathe in the color red, and visualize red filling that space. Silently repeat the mantra "Lam" while you exhale. Continue this for a couple of minutes.

Now move to the second chakra, below the navel. Breathe in the color orange, and visualize orange filling that space. Silently repeat the mantra "Vam" while you exhale. Continue this for a couple of minutes. Now move to the third chakra, at the solar plexus. Breathe in the color yellow and visualize yellow filling that space. Silently repeat the mantra "Ram" while you exhale. Continue this for a couple of minutes.

Now move to the fourth chakra, at the heart center. Breathe in the color green and visualize green filling that space. Silently repeat the mantra "Yam" while you exhale. Continue this for a couple of minutes.

Now move to the fifth chakra, at the middle of the throat. Breathe in the color blue and visualize blue filling that space. Silently repeat the mantra "Hum" while you exhale. Continue this for a couple of minutes.

Now move to the sixth chakra, at the third eye. Breathe in the color indigo and visualize indigo filling that space. Silently repeat the mantra "Ksham" while you exhale. Continue this for a couple of minutes.

Now move to the seventh chakra, at the crown of the head. Breathe in the color violet and visualize violet filling that space. Silently repeat the mantra "Om" while you exhale. Continue this for a couple of minutes.

Now take some time to relax more deeply, and visually surround yourself in white light. Feel the light permeating your being and radiating from you at the same time.

Breathe and become aware of your surroundings before slowly opening your eyes. Stretch a little before going on with your activities.

For more information about meditation, including downloadable guided meditations, visit my site: PSMeditation.com.

⟡ DAILY PRACTICES ⟡

We live, in fact, in a world starved for solitude,
silence, and private: and therefore starved
for meditation and true friendship.
– C.S. Lewis

I think we can all feel the uncertainty in the air, the trepidation, and conflicting viewpoints. This is a difficult time for the world, and we can't help but pick up on these energies and feel it within ourselves. So, what do we do? What can we do?

There is so much information out there. We see it on our computers and television sets, read about it in the paper... and it is good to stay informed. We need to know what is going on. We need to be able to make good decisions. But we can't make good decisions when we are coming from a place of fear. We need to keep some balance in our lives so that we can make decisions and take action coming from a place of centeredness and calm.

In-form-ation is "in form" or in body – representing the physical world. Information is all around us in abundance, we see it all the time! What we need to do now is to shift our attention to spirit – to seek "in-spir-ation!" Inspiration is all around us as well, but the information is shouting so loudly at us right now that we can't hear it. The only way we can tune in is to spend some time in silence. In that silence we will find our peace.

Knowing that there is a Divine Plan at work may offer us some comfort. Even with all of our concerns and worries, there comes a point when we must turn our troubles over to God, and know that right action is taking place. We don't know what is going to happen, or how things are going to turn out, but through our spiritual studies we have learned that somehow, someway, everything happens exactly the way it is supposed to. Our minds may be in turmoil trying to process the politics of it all, but our hearts remind us to have faith.

So, once again it all comes down to our spiritual practices. The good that we do for ourselves is good that we do for the world. Our own growth helps the world to expand, and to open up to the possibilities that abound. We are all in this together, and individually we can each make a difference right where we are. These practices can become healthy habits, that we look forward to, and that sustain us through whatever stresses come our way. Throughout these trying times, let's do our best to maintain inner peace. This is our contribution; this is our responsibility.

Throughout the day, carve out a little time to remember what is really important. We all get caught up in the trivia of life, and we often let time get eaten up with things that don't really matter to us. No matter how much time we have, we can use it mindfully. This is our choice to make!

Look deep into nature,
and then you will understand everything better.
– Albert Einstein

MAKING THE MOST OF YOUR ALONE TIME, WHEN YOU HAVE:

∘≪ 5 MINUTES ≫∘

- Bliss out! Close your eyes, rest your head, put your feet up and breathe!

- Spend five minutes in peace and quiet – no talking, no reading, no listening – just CALM. Sit and just "be.

- "Dance like no one's watching!" Crank up your favorite CD and go nuts. Let the energy flow from your fingers to your toes!

- Cuddle your kitty cat. Studies have shown that stroking pets reduces stress and lowers blood pressure.

- Repeat an affirmation. Maybe it's a quote you live by, or a goal you're trying to reach – give it your undivided attention and remind yourself just how important that is to you.

- Go through your calendar and see what events you've got coming up. Schedule in some time to get ready so you're not feeling ambushed when the big days arrive!

- Give yourself a massage! Use a rich cream to moisturize your hands and massage them thoroughly. Apply extra to elbows, knees and those tired tootsies.

∘≪ 30 MINUTES ≫∘

- Spend time in nature. Do we ever get outdoors enough anymore? Go for your own nature walk. Notice the flowers, the leaves, the birds – ah, this beautiful planet is paradise!

- Write a letter. Is this a lost art or what? Not an e-mail letter, but a real, old-fashioned pen and paper kind of a thing! Send it to your favorite aunt or grandmother – they'll love it!

- Organize your photos. They have been piling up, haven't they? Whether you have copies in a drawer or dozens stored on your hard drive that haven't been printed out, find a way to make use of these moments caught on camera. Slip them into an album, or start a scrapbook. You'll be so happy to have the saved memories later on.

- Give yourself a mani-pedi. A little primping will make you feel all new.

- Meditate. This is the best, healthiest thing you can do for yourself. Clear your mind, close your eyes, and focus on your breath. Whenever thoughts come to disturb the tranquility, see them drift by like a cloud, and go back to watching your breath.

☞ HALF A DAY ☜

- Take yourself on a date! See that movie that you've been dying to see and couldn't drag your friends to. Bring a picnic to the park and play on the swings. Do what YOU want to do, but never give yourself permission to.

- Clean out your closet. Challenge yourself to fill up bags to give to charity. Be ruthless with your stuff this time. If you don't love it, lose it!

- Read a book. Really. Just for the FUN of it. Nothing that is assigned, nothing you have to analyze or write a paper about. Whether it's Jane Austen or Jackie Collins, just enjoy reading for reading's sake.

- Write out your life's story. Someday your grandkids will ask about what life was like as a teen way back in the 2000's – you can get out your journal and tell them just what was on your mind! Think about what moments stand out in your memory, and why.

- Experiment in the kitchen. Have you ever made your own pie crust? A soufflé? Want to try? Now's the time. You've got the place to yourself, no one to look over your shoulder – so go for it!

- Luxuriate! Take a bubble bath, light candles, take time doing your hair. Pamper yourself.

☞ A WHOLE DAY ☜

- Take a field trip. How many sites are there right in your city that you've never seen? Go out and explore. Visit a museum, try a new restaurant, get out a map and go.

- Make a multi-media presentation. Start with your digital camera or video camera. Decide on a topic, your life, your interests, etc. Shoot a bunch of footage and come up with commentary. Put it all together into a computer program like Power Point and you've got your own little piece of history preserved.

- Redecorate! Make over your room entirely. A fresh coat of paint in a brilliant new color will certainly pep up your space. Shop for some inexpensive fabric to recover your old bedspread – whip up some simple throw pillow using no-sew fabric glue. Kick out the clutter and make a display of your collectibles. Have fun re-purposing items you don't use. Move furniture around and give yourself a whole new perspective.

- Get creative. Drop by one of those paint-your-own-pottery places and personalize a platter for parents' anniversary. Pull out your old sketch book and pretend you're in Paris. Ride your bike to some beautiful scenery for inspiration and draw until your heart's content.

- Start making a list of all the things you want to do, and then start doing them every time you get a little bit of alone time.

◦⊷ FEEL THE BLISS! ⊶◦

If a person's basic state of mind is serene and calm,
then it is possible for this inner peace to overwhelm
a painful physical experience.
– The Dalai Lama

I think you can see from this list that spirituality is all about being joyful. This is our natural state of being. When we are balanced, when we are unaffected by stress, when we are at our best, we are open to experiencing the bliss. We have access to it at all times. The Dalai Lama, one of the most spiritual people on the planet, is an excellent example of this. Of course this man has a lot of stress, political and otherwise, but whenever you see him, he has a big smile on his face. He giggles like a little kid. He exudes bliss. Enlightenment is about lightening up. We don't have to take ourselves too seriously. When we know who we are, we know what is important in life.

So that brings up the big question: "Who Am I?"

As we start spending more time in silence, more time in nature, more time mindfully going about our activities, the answer becomes clearer. We are more than our bodies. We are more than the roles we play. And so is everyone else. We are all connected, and intertwined in each other's lives. This recognition allows us to open up the scope of our vision and to see and experience more of the unlimited possibilities that are available to us at all times. And that automatically brings us bliss.

CHAPTER 7

WEIGHT MANAGEMENT

One word frees us of all the weight
and pain in life. That word is love.
– Sophocles

☞ CRAVINGS AS CLUES ☜

A big part of controlling our weight is controlling our cravings. We have these cravings and we want to eat, and that's when we often overeat, and then gain weight. Our cravings can be a factor of an imbalance in our doshas. When we discover the imbalance, we can work on that, reducing the cravings and feeling better all around.

- The craving for comfort foods indicates a Vata imbalance. Comfort foods are sweet, creamy, carbohydrate-heavy foods. This is really a signal that our body wants something warm, nurturing, calming or grounding to balance out an excess of Vata. We can achieve this with Vata pacifying techniques: drink Vata tea, use aromatherapy (vanilla, orange), hug a friend, or listen to your favorite music.

The craving for salty foods indicates a Pitta imbalance. We crave salty foods like chips, pretzels and nuts, when we feel frustrated, angry, excited or annoyed. To balance out Pitta, drink Pitta tea, use aromatherapy (sandalwood, mint), walk in the moonlight, or look at beautiful landscaping or artwork.

The craving for caffeine, or chocolate, indicates a Kapha imbalance. Kaphas need something stimulating to overcome feelings of lethargy or depression. Instead of downing coffee, cola or candy bars, implement some Kapha pacifying techniques: drink Kapha tea, use aromatherapy (spicy scents like rosemary and clove), or dance around to some lively music.

The Ayurvedic approach to weight control is very simple and straightforward. Kapha types tend to have the most trouble with weight imbalance. Kaphas have a slower metabolism, so they are more prone to weight gain. Kapha is made up of earth and water, so to boost metabolism one strategy is to increase the fire element. Flavor foods with spicy spices like pepper, ginger and curries. Eat foods that are easy to digest: warm, light and cooked. Nothing fried, and avoid dairy and sugar.

Pittas can also have issues with weight gain, which is usually caused when digestive enzymes are out of whack and there is too much acid. In this case there is an abundance of fire, so spicy foods are not good. Instead, what Pittas can do to improve this condition is to eat three meals a day. Sweet, juicy fruits like pears and peaches are great for Pittas, as are licorice and fennel seed. Pittas also need to be sure to get to bed before 10 pm, when Pitta time kicks in and they get the munchies.

When Vata types gain weight it is usually due to stress and emotional eating. To reduce stress, it is important for Vatas to meditate twice a day and to keep a regular routine. Vatas also need to remember to eat warm, cooked meals in a relaxed atmosphere and to not rush through their meals.

AYURVEDA AND WEIGHT MANAGEMENT
KAPHA

Most often weight gain is caused by a slow metabolism. This is common for a person who is a classic Kapha type. Kapha dosha is comprised of the earth and water elements, so this type of individual will reflect those qualities. A Kapha person will be structurally bigger, with bigger bones and a more easy-going, stable, gentle personality.

For a Kapha person, being skinny is usually not a healthy goal. If you are prone to gain weight, and are always five to ten pounds overweight no matter how little you eat, it would go against your nature to ever be really thin. Rather, it would be better to balance your metabolism, increase your ability to digest sugars and carbohydrates by adopting a Kapha balancing diet and lifestyle, and allow your body to naturally find its ideal weight. You may not be skinny, you may always weigh five to ten pounds more than average, but you will feel better and look healthier, and you will lose most of your excess weight.

☞ DIET ☜

The main principle for balancing Kapha is to introduce some of the fire element into your food and lifestyle. This will balance the earthen and watery elements of Kapha dosha. Bring on the spicy! Flavor your vegetables and soups with spices that are mildly pungent, such as black pepper, fresh ginger, and turmeric

Other tastes to balance Kapha dosha are the bitter and astringent tastes. These include green leafy vegetables, split mung dahl and other bean soups, and astringent vegetables such as broccoli, cauliflower and Brussels sprouts. It's important to cook your vegetables and eat them warm, rather than relying on raw vegetables. Raw vegetables are difficult to digest, so to balance Kapha dosha you want to eat warm, light, cooked foods.

Quinoa is an excellent grain for managing weight, as it has high protein and zinc content (4 mg of zinc per cup). But it should be cooked with a bit of ghee or olive oil, as otherwise it may be too drying.

Basmati rice is also a good grain for Kapha dosha, because it has a more drying quality than other types of rice. Quinoa is even better because it has the intelligence of fire to support weight loss.

The fire element can even be added to the water you drink. If you boil your water for five minutes on the stove, you are adding the intelligence of fire to your drinking water. If you sip the water throughout the day, this energy will permeate the molecules of water, and thus permeate your body. You won't notice anything right away, but if you continue with this routine, in time you will feel less fatigue. This is because Kapha dosha tends to create a feeling of lethargy, and by introducing the fire element in the water, you'll gradually feel more energetic.

If you are Kapha by nature, you'll want to stay away from heavy, cold desserts such as ice cream and cheesecake, as these will only slow your metabolism and increase the cold, heavy qualities of Kapha in your body. Rich desserts, fried foods, foods made with refined sugar and refined flour, cold foods and drinks — all of these should be avoided if you want to balance Kapha and your weight.

EXERCISE

Regular exercise is the most important change you can make to improve your metabolism. For Kaphas it's a good idea to exercise every day, to the point of breaking a sweat. People with excessive Kapha dosha often feel somewhat complacent or even lethargic, and they might have to push themselves a little to exercise every day. Usually Kapha types need more vigorous exercise for a longer period to have the same effect as milder exercise would have on a Vata person. Running, weight lifting, any aerobic or cardio-vascular exercise is good for Kaphas. This helps them to have more energy, to feel motivated and stimulated.

BREATHING

Even making a habit of breathing more deeply can help charge the metabolism with more of the fire element. When Kapha dosha is out of balance, one of the first things that happens is that the person becomes a shallow breather. Deeper breathing is healthy for all body types, but especially for Kapha dosha, because deeper breathing helps wake up the body's metabolism. When the metabolism is lower and breathing is shallow, the body's channels get blocked and cause even more lethargy, which becomes a vicious cycle.

Don't try to force your breathing, but just easily make a habit of breathing more deeply. It's a good idea to learn pranayama, the yogic breathing exercise that prepares the mind and body for meditation. These gentle exercises cultivate deeper breathing and help cleanse the pathways of prana, or life breath, in the body, removing obstructions and enhancing metabolism.

❖ WHEN TO EAT ❖

Everyone, and especially those of us with more Kapha dosha in our physiology, need to be sure to eat our main meal when the sun is strongest, right at noon. This is because the body's internal digestive fire, called agni, is also strongest at noon. If you eat your main meal then, you'll digest it more easily and create less of the waste product of digestion, the toxic ama, which blocks the channels and slows metabolism.

The digestive fire is weaker first thing in the morning and in the evening before bed, so breakfast and dinner should be lighter meals. An ideal breakfast for balancing metabolism for all three body-types is a cooked apple or pear with cooked prunes and figs. This breakfast choice is light and sustains most people until the lunch hour, between noon and one p.m., when we can eat our heaviest meal. A healthy dinner for Kaphas might be soup made with vegetables, grains and beans and flavored with spices such as cumin, fresh ginger, black pepper, and turmeric. You can mix your own spices, or use Kapha Churna, a spice blend specifically formulated for balancing Kapha. Kitchari, made with rice and split mung dahl, is also a light Kapha-pacifying meal.

Be Trim Herbal Tea from MAPI is an excellent formula for enhancing metabolism of carbohydrates and sugar. Be Trim Tea also helps to curb cravings and false hunger pangs.

∞ THE KAPHA DIET ∞

	FAVOR	REDUCE/AVOID
QUALITIES	Light, dry, warm, cooked	Heavy, oily, cold
TASTES	Pungent, bitter, astringent	Sweet, sour, salty
QUANTITIES	Small – do not overeat	
DAIRY	Warm low-fat or nonfat milk	All other
SWEETENERS	Honey	All others
OILS	Small amounts only: almond, corn, ghee, safflower, sunflower	All except for small amounts of oils listed
GRAINS	Barley, corn, millet, rye	Oats, wheat
FRUITS	Light, dry fruits: apple, apricot, cranberry, dried fruits, pear, pomegranate	Heavy, juicy, sweet, sour: avocado, banana, coconut, date, fig, grapefruit, grape, mango, melon, orange, papaya, peach, pineapple, plum
VEGETABLES	All okay except those listed	Sweet, juicy vegetable: cucumber, sweet potato, tomato
SPICES	All okay except salt	Salt
NUTS/SEEDS	Pumpkin seeds, sunflower seeds	All others
BEANS	All okay except tofu	Tofu
MEATS	Poultry (white meat), white meat fish (except shellfish)	Red meat, shellfish

AYURVEDA AND WEIGHT MANAGEMENT
VATA

Those who are Vata dominant, are normally thin and wiry. But that does not mean weight gain is never a problem. Sometimes Vata types are thin all their lives and then suddenly put on weight because their metabolism changes. Vatas are susceptible to mental stress because they tend to overuse their minds thinking, worrying, planning, problem-solving. When under stress they also tend to forget to eat regularly, thus disturbing their digestion, and creating ama. This often leads to weight gain.

❧ ROUTINE ❧

Those dominant in Vata need to stick to a regular routine, to balance the uneven, variable nature of Vata dosha. It's important that they go to bed early, well before ten o'clock and rise early, before 6 a.m. A regular routine with a good night's sleep is one of the best ways to keep Vata in balance. Regular meals are essential, with three warm, cooked meals a day. It's important to eat them at the same time every day, as Vata digestion tends to be irregular. By eating at the same time, your digestive enzymes will prepare to digest the food and digestion will be stronger. Avoid work that is stressful to the mind, and practice relaxing exercise such as yoga and pranayama (breathing exercises). Abhyanga, a daily oil massage is especially important for Vata, and there are specially blended oils with herbs that help to alleviate the dry skin that is often a result of Vata imbalance. The skin is one of the primary seats of Vata dosha in the body, so massaging your body every morning with warm, Vata-pacifying oil can go a long way toward soothing your entire nervous system and emotions. The more relaxed you are, and the more regular your routine, the better you will withstand day-to-day stress and the less likely you are to fall prey to weight imbalances.

Many times people with Vata imbalances find themselves in a rush, always in a hurry. It's not healthy for anyone to always be rushing around, to constantly have to hurry, and it's especially harmful to people with Vata imbalances. If you find yourself in that situation, it's important to cultivate a habit of taking it easy and slowing down. Learn to structure a more relaxed, mellow daily routine. This is important for mental, emotional and physical health.

❧ DIET ❧

When a Vata imbalance is the underlying cause of a weight problem, it's important to eat a balanced diet that is easy to digest but also nurturing. Take the middle path, and eat a tridoshic diet, which means one that balances all three doshas. Avoid foods that are too hot and spicy (such as food spiced with chilies, cayenne, and black mustard seed), and at the same time avoid foods that are ice cold, such as ice cream, iced drinks, and cold, heavy desserts. Stay away from foods that are too heavy (such as aged cheeses, meats, and heavy desserts) and also avoid foods that are too light and dry, such as crackers, cold cereals, and packaged snacks. In general, avoid leftovers; frozen, canned or packaged foods, and processed foods of all kinds.

Eat foods that are fresh, organic, and whole. Favor foods that transform easily into ojas, the product of perfect digestion that improves immunity, bliss and happiness in the body, rather than ama. For breakfast try stewed apples and pears. Cooking these fruits so that they are warm, and adding a little sweetness with ghee makes them much more digestible. For dinner eat whole grains and soups made with fresh vegetables. And for the main meal at lunchtime include organic vegetables such as zucchini and loki squash, grains such as quinoa, and light proteins such as split mung bean. Cook with light, nourishing oils such as ghee and olive oil.

❧ EXERCISE ❧

Because Vatas don't have this huge reserve of energy, too much exercise will just wear them out. They do need movement, and activity, but they don't need the kind of strenuous exercise that a Kapha person needs. Vatas do best with yoga, walking, dancing, and Pilates.

❧ HERBS ❧

Herbs that help with mental stress include Ashwagandha and Arjuna. Ashwagandha is an adaptogenic, which means that it helps alleviate the physical fatigue that leads to a sense of mental "dullness." Brahmi is an herb famous for reducing stress and anxiety. These herbs are used in Worry Free tablets from Maharishi Ayurveda Products, or you can purchase them individually in health food stores. Emotional stress is another cause of weight gain, particularly in Vata types. Arjuna is known to support both the physical and emotional heart, and is a key ingredient in MAPI's Blissful Joy tablets.

⊶⊰ THE VATA DIET ⊱⊶

	FAVOR	REDUCE/AVOID
QUALITIES	Heavy, warm, cooked	Light, cold, dry, raw
TASTES	Sweet, sour, salty	Bitter, pungent, astringent
QUANTITIES	Larger portions okay	
DAIRY	All dairy okay, look for dairy alternatives when possible	
SWEETENERS	All okay in moderation	
OILS	All okaya	
GRAINS	Rice, wheat, cooked oats	Barley, corn, millet, rye
FRUITS	Sweet, sour and juicy fruits: avocado, banana, berry, cherry, grape, mango, melon, orange, peaches, plum, pineapple	Light, dry fruits: uncooked apple, cranberry, dried fruits, pears, pomegranate
VEGETABLES	Most vegetables in moderation when cooked, especially: Asparagus, beet, carrot, green beans, okra, sweet potato	Uncooked vegetables, cabbage, sprouts
SPICES	Sweet, heating spices are best, other spices in moderation	Large quantities of bitter, pungent or astringent spices: chili, coriander, fenugreek, parsley, saffron, turmeric
NUTS/SEEDS	All okay, almonds especially good	
BEANS	Garbanzos, red lentils, mung beans, tofu	All other beans except those listed
MEATS	Chicken, turkey, seafood	Red meat

WEIGHT MANAGEMENT
PITTA

Since Pitta is associated with the fire element, it would seem that a person with high Pitta would not have any problem burning up carbohydrates and sugars. Yet if the person doesn't take care of the digestion, there can be problems. For example, if someone with a lot of Pitta skips breakfast or another meal, that can create ama, digestive impurities, because the digestive fire becomes too strong. With too much fire, stomach acids can "burn" the food and even damage the stomach.

To understand how this happens, think of setting an empty pot on the stove. The heat is on, but there's nothing to cook. Instead, the pot itself gets burned. In the same way, if you have a strong digestive fire but you don't feed it regularly, then the digestive enzymes go out of balance, burn the food and create ama the next time you eat.

Many people with high Pitta dosha are overweight, precisely because they are not eating regularly and as a result ama has coated their digestive system. When ama blocks the channels of digestion and the channels that circulate nutrients throughout the body, then metabolism slows down and weight gain results.

In this case, the added factor of hyperacidity creates additional problems, because the Pitta type's fiery digestion tries to overcompensate for the ama and blocked channels by producing more acidity. We could take an over-the-counter antacid, but still gain weight because the body is now clogged with ama. The antacid worked on the symptom, but not the cause of the symptom.

When this happens, it's a good idea to consult an Ayurvedic practitioner for specific recommendations, because it is important to repair the pot first, so to speak, and stop the damage to the stomach area from excess digestive acids.

⌖⤛ DIET ⤜⌖
Pitta people need to get into the habit of eating three meals a day, starting with breakfast. This is very important, because without food the stomach will continue to be burned by digestive acids. Eating a cooked apple or pears with cooked prunes or figs for breakfast soothes the digestive fire without overloading it. Raw pears or other sweet, juicy fruits also help to balance Pitta. Cooked oatmeal is also a good breakfast for Pitta types. A vegetable that is good for weight management is daikon radish.

This white radish can be grated and added to dahl or soups for a mildly spicy flavor. Include sweet vegetables for lunch and dinner, such as squashes that are white inside (zucchini, loki or yellow squash). Steam them well and then sauté them in ghee with mild, cooling spices such as powdered fennel, a little bit of cumin and a little bit of turmeric. You can add one or two whole cloves to dahl, soup, vegetables or grains as you cook them, because even though clove seems to be pungent and sharp, it actually has a cooling effect if you cook with it but don't chew it. Make sure you get the whole cloves out before serving – or grind the cloves before cooking with them.

Mung bean is a good source of protein when cooked as a soup with spices. Quinoa and basmati rice, cooked with a little olive oil or ghee, are recommended grains to balance Pitta. It might seem counter-intuitive to add oils into cooking when weight is an issue, but remember that in the case of a Pitta imbalance, often the stomach has been damaged by hyperacidity. So healthy fats such as ghee and olive oil will lubricate the area and help repair the damage. Flavor foods with Pitta Churna, a delicious spice blend specifically created for balancing Pitta. Pitta Tea is ideal to help balance Pitta.

Pittas need to avoid those pungent spices such as chilies, cayenne, and black mustard seed; these increase acidity. It would seem like heavy, cold, or sweet foods would cool the acidity. But in reality heavy, cold foods will only make the acidity problem worse by creating more ama and blocking the channels of digestion and metabolism. It's better to cool the digestive fire by cooking with cooling spices, and by eating light desserts with our meal such as fruit crisps. Just a little sweet to balance all that hot and spicy that comes naturally to Pittas!

Cool, but not ice cold, drinks help to keep Pitta in balance. The idea is to calm that fire, but not put it out completely. Avoid carbonated drinks which tend to disrupt digestion. Choose sweet fruit juices and pure water to stay hydrated. Pitta tea is delicious chilled! The Pitta diet calls for more sweet, bitter and astringent tastes. Salads with leafy greens are a great way to get these tastes in. Cooling spices, such as mint, fennel, and anise can be added to foods.

⟡ EXERCISE ⟡

Pittas are very competitive, so it's great for them to get involved in sporting activities. If it's running, they'll want to best their time on the track. If it's a team sport, they'll want to go out and play, and probably want to be the captain of the team! Pittas do well on a schedule. They're very organized, so to have a regular appointment to workout, or to have a game, works well with their personality. Swimming and water sports are cooling, so these are ideal for balancing Pitta. And Pittas tend to enjoy skiing and snowboarding as well.

⌖⊛ SLEEP ⊛⌖

Ayurveda recommends that everyone, and particularly people who are predominantly Pitta, should go to sleep before the Pitta time of the evening (10:00 p.m. to 2:00 a.m.). Even if you feel like you have a lot of energy then, or feel more creative. It's not a good idea to stay awake during the Pitta time of night, because this only aggravates Pitta dosha further. After 10 you will likely get that "second wind" and find it harder to fall asleep. And, you will probably get hungry and thirsty and may just eat that stash of packaged cookies or salty snacks, or drink soft drinks or alcohol. All of these bad habits just aggravate Pitta dosha more and contribute to weight gain.

⚬❊ THE PITTA DIET ❊⚬

	FAVOR	REDUCE/AVOID
QUALITIES	Cool or warm, liquid	Hot
TASTES	Sweet, bitter, astringent	Salty, sour, pungent
QUANTITIES	Moderate portions	
DAIRY	Butter, ghee, lassi, milk	Cheese, butter-milk, sour cream, yogurt (except lassi)
SWEETENERS	All okay except those listed	Honey, molasses
OILS	Coconut, olive, soy, sunflower	Almond, corn, safflower, sesame
GRAINS	Barley, oats, wheat, white rice	Corn millet, brown rice, rye
FRUITS	Sweet, ripe fruits: apple, avocado, cherry, fig, mango, melon, pear, pomegranate, prune, raisin	Sour, unripe fruits: apricot, banana, berry, cranberry, grapefruit, olive, papaya, peach, persimmon
VEGETABLES	Asparagus, bell peppers, broccoli, Brussels sprouts, cabbage, cauliflower, celery, cucumber, green bean, okra, peas, potato, sprouts, squash, all leafy greens except spinach	Beets, carrot, chili, eggplant, garlic, onion, radish, spinach, tomato
SPICES	Sweet, bitter, astringent spices: cardamom, cilantro, cinnamon, coriander, dill, fennel, mint, saffron	Pungent, heating spices, especially chili
NUTS/SEEDS	Coconut, pumpkin seeds, sunflower seeds	All others
BEANS	Garbanzo, mung, soybean, tofu	All others
MEATS	Chicken, egg whites, turkey, shrimp	Egg yolks, red meat

❧❧ BREATHING EXERCISES ❧❧

"Prana" in Sanskrit means "breath." In Vedic texts, prana is recognized as the energy of spiritual light, and this is the substance of our subtle body. Prana is an energy that can be transferred from one person to another through various hands-on treatments like massage. We energize our prana through meditation, yoga, mantra practice, and by eating nutritious foods. Another way to work on our prana is through "pranayama" or yogic breathing exercises.

We all need breath to survive. Even plants breathe. And even though this appears to be a kind of mechanical process, one we don't really think about, Ayurveda explains that the whole process of inhaling and exhaling is full of life itself. Notice how the breath changes when our emotions come into play. When we are scared, we tense up, and hold our breath, and our breathing is irregular. When we are happy, and laughing, we breathe deeply, our breathing is rhythmic. Pranayama translated means "to control the breath." By doing so, we are helping to settle and control our busy minds.

Pranayama is often considered to be an art, and some people consider it to be an important part of their spiritual practice. Our bodies are made up of pairs of things: two arms, two legs, two lungs, two nostrils, and even two brains, left and right. Pranayama helps us to even out the balance of energy on both sides, including our Shiva and Shakti, male and female energy. This brings us to a greater sense of awareness.

There are many different types of pranayama, but let's look at just three:

1. ***Alternate Nostril Breathing Pranayama.***
   This exercise is good for all three doshas.
   - Begin by sitting with your back straight. Be comfortable, either on the floor or in a chair.
   - Take your right hand thumb, and with it, close your right nostril.
   - Inhale through your left nostril, deep into the diaphragm. Hold it for a moment.
   - Close your left nostril with the ring finger of your right hand.
   - Exhale through your right nostril. Hold it a moment.
   - Inhale through your right nostril. Hold it a moment.
   - Close your right nostril with your right thumb and begin the sequence again.

You can do this exercise for 8-10 "rounds" and will notice an increase in your energy level, and feel like you have a clearer mind.

2. **Cooling Pranayama**

    This exercise is particularly good for Pittas.

    - Curl your tongue into a tube shape and stick it out a little. If you can't curl your tongue, then part your lips, keeping your teeth together, and put your tongue up against your teeth.
    - Inhale through your mouth, allowing the air to pass over your tongue.
    - Draw your tongue in and close your mouth.
    - Swallow.
    - Exhale through the nose, keeping the mouth closed.

3. **Breath of Fire Pranayama**

    This exercise is good for both Vatas and Kaphas.

    - Inhale gently through the nose.
    - Exhale through the nose more actively, with more strength, almost like you're blowing something out your nose.
    - Inhale gently again.
    - Blow out through the nose again.
    - Start out slowly, and then gradually increase your speed. The idea is to sound like a train moving slowly at first, and then picking up speed. Practice one round of 20-30 exhales, then rest for a minute or so. You can practice up to five rounds at a time, twice a day.

CHAPTER 8

THE 28 - DAY PROGRAM

Health is a state of complete physical, mental and social
well-being, and not merely the absence
of disease or infirmity.
– World Health Organization, 1948

The Perfect Balance Diet is all about getting ourselves into really good habits. To do this we have to take action. We have to make a commitment and stick to it. Like any change, it might be awkward or uncomfortable at first. We might have a dozen excuses as to why we can't, won't or shouldn't embark on this challenge to bring ourselves back into balance. But in our hearts we know what is good for us. We know that it just takes a subtle shift to make everything in our lives fall into place. So we're ready.

Mark out 28 consecutive days that you will commit to stay on The Perfect Balance Diet program. This new routine, and the exercises that go along with it, will not interfere with your day – on the contrary, it will enhance it. Don't worry about counting calories, about getting on the scale, about portion control. Just follow the guidelines for the ideal ayurvedic routine (below), for eating the ayurvedic way for weight management (Chapter 7), for improved digestion (Chapter 2) and for meditation (Chapter 6). You will know the difference this program makes in your life by the way you feel. You will have more energy; you will feel lighter, and more light-hearted. If you want to measure weight loss, then weigh yourself on Day 1, and again on Day 28. But in between, don't even think about it!

You can start this program anytime – even right now! If you want to be in harmony with nature and have that extra boost of support, you might want to try starting the program near the time of the new moon, which signifies new beginnings. If you have a job that you go to Monday through Fridays, you might want to start the program on a Sunday, so that you can use the extra time to prepare for the week ahead by grocery shopping and organizing a bit.

Just as the seasons have a routine that they follow, nature expresses itself throughout each day in consistent, predictable way. To be in harmony with nature, to allow nature to work with us, we can ride along with this flow of energy.

At sunrise, or about 6:00 A.M., we are at the end of Vata time and the beginning of Kapha time. It is best to awaken by 6:00 A.M. before Kapha kicks into full gear and you feel so relaxed that you don't want to get out of bed. On awakening, you feel slow, relaxed, calm: all Kapha attributes. Kapha lasts until about 10:00 A.M. During this time is when you prepare for your day. Meditation, exercise, massage, shower, breakfast and then starting work.

From 10:00 A.M. to 2:00 P.M., it is Pitta time. You are at your most active and efficient during these hours, so it's the best time to work. At noon, or lunchtime, your appetite is at its peak. Eat lunch between noon and 1:00 P.M. to use Pitta to your advantage. Lunch also should be your largest meal of the day. Of course, because of our western culture, this is not always possible. However we can be mindful and choose foods that are wholesome, fresh, and beneficial. It's also important to eat at approximately the same time each day so that the body can prepare itself for the work it needs to do digesting. By eating our largest meal at this time we are giving ourselves the whole rest of the day to adequately digest and assimilate our food.

From 2:00 P.M. to 6:00 P.M. is Vata time, when you are most alert and creative. It's a good time to brainstorm, come up with new ideas, and work on problem solving. A light dinner should be eaten before 6:00 P.M. if possible to take advantage of this energy.

The cycle repeats again in the evening hours. From 6:00 P.M. to 10:00 P.M. is Kapha time. Sunset brings the body rest and a slower pace. It is best to get to bed by 10:00 P.M. to take advantage of the natural Kapha rhythm of this time. For best digestion, eat dinner at least three hours before bedtime. Those who require more sleep, younger children, teens, some Vata types or those in the Vata time of life, should go to bed earlier so that they will still arise at sunrise. Those who require less sleep, like some Kaphas, should still go to bed at 10 pm, and then wake up earlier in the morning.

Pitta time is 10:00 P.M. to 2:00 A.M., when Pitta keeps the body warm; the body also uses the Pitta heat to digest food and rebuild body tissues. This is when we get our most restorative sleep. When we go to bed later than 10 P.M. we are missing out on this. Because Pitta makes us mentally active, it's also more difficult to get to sleep if we are in bed later than 10 P.M.

Vata time occurs again at 2:00 A.M. to 6:00 A.M. Vata creativity is expressed as active dreams. At this time, brain impulses are at their most active for the night. We use this time to subconsciously problem-solve.

◦◈ THE AYURVEDIC DAILY CLOCK ◈◦

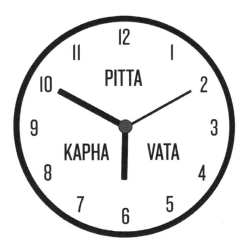

The Ideal Ayurvedic Routine follows. This routine is what you do everyday, for sure, for the entire 28 days. In addition, I have provided some suggested activities for each individual day. The days are broken up into four weeks. The first week we will focus on our surroundings, getting our environment into a place that support us and our efforts. The second week we will pay attention more to our physical body, and getting in tune what we need to do to take care of ourselves. The third week is all about the mind. We'll take a more intellectual approach to this whole process and explore our creativity. And the fourth week we will embrace the spirit.

By the end of the 28 days you'll have a new outlook, and a new look! How you feel on the inside definitely shows in how you look on the outside. People will be commenting on the change – they may even notice it before you do.

Ideal daily Ayurvedic Routine:

- Wake up at sunrise, about 6:00 A.M.

- Use the bathroom.

- Brush your teeth and tongue.

- Give yourself an Ayurvedic massage (Abhyanga – see detailed instructions below).

- Do your Yoga stretches and/or your exercise program for your dosha.

- Take a warm shower or bath.

- Meditate (Ideally 20-30 minutes).

- Eat a light breakfast based on your dosha.

- Work or study.

- Eat lunch, your largest meal of the day, at the same time each day, between noon and 1:00 P.M.

- Work or study.

- Meditate before dinner.

- Eat a light dinner, at the same time each day, preferably before 6:30 P.M.

- Take a short walk to aid digestion.

- Relax. Read. Listen to music. Visit with friends.

- Get to bed by 10:00 P.M.

If your mornings are hectic and you need to leave the house very early, you may choose to do your massage and shower in the evening. Doing so will give you an especially restful night's sleep. If you wake up hungry, as many of us do, you may choose to eat breakfast before your shower. Ayurveda will prove beneficial in whatever way it is blended into your routine. Even just adding a couple of new things into your established routine will give you a good start. There are no hard and fast rules here. Be gentle, and flexible with yourself and use this as a good guideline.

Consistency is what matters, and what will make the biggest difference. It is nice to take your time in the morning and fit in all of the Ayurvedic routine, but if you are in a hurry, it is better to do it all quickly rather than to skip it altogether. And be easy on yourself. Ayurveda is flexible, so figure out what works for you. You might not be able to do every single thing at first, but if you can do more than half, you will still see benefits. The main thing is not to stress about it. Start where you are comfortable, and grow from there.

◦◦◦ MOVEMENT ◦◦◦

A big part of this holistic plan for Perfect Balance is movement. Movement is natural for us – we are designed for movement, to get from one place to another using our own energy.

The word "exercise" seems unnatural to us. Perhaps because we're not moving enough, we feel the need to impose movement upon our bodies to stay in shape and maintain our state of balance. Somehow when we were young we could just go out and play and that would be exercise enough. But somewhere down the line we got stuck behind our desks and now we have to schedule in time to "work out." Work sounds much more tedious than play, doesn't it?

So let's change our mind-set. Instead of working out, getting some exercise, let's go play! Let's revel in all types of movement that gets our bodies in tune with our potential. After all, when we are moving our bodies we are sending fresh blood and oxygen to all of our organs – it is the whole body that feels the benefits of movement.

Think about all the types of movement that appeal to you. Morning stretches in bed can help you to wake up. A walk in the sunshine helps to keep you grounded throughout the day. After sitting at a desk, and being on the computer for an extended period of time, it feels good to do some yoga poses, and shoulder openers, some you can do right from your chair.

In the theme of going out to play – I love to skip! It sounds silly, but it is much more appealing to me than running. My friend Kim "Skipper" Corbin started a website www.iskip.com that has gotten a skipping movement underway. I have to admit, sometimes when I see someone coming the other direction, doing a jog or power walk, I start to walk. But then I think – how is this any different than any other kind of movement? The only difference I can see is that I'm having fun! Whether we're strapping wheels to our feet to rollerblade, or jumping up and down on a trampoline, we're making use of our bodies.

There's a park by our home, and I also love to go swing on the swings. Sometimes I have to wait for my turn if there are kids there. But I love when kids are there because it reminds me of the childlike quality with which we can approach movement. We don't need to stress about how well we are doing with any particular movement; we just need to move! And in this movement we are actually celebrating our lives, our connection with the earth, and our place upon the planet. We can skip and dance and twirl down the street if we feel like it!

Yoga is a wonderful way to move the body because there are so many different accommodations, or variations, depending our your level of fitness. It doesn't matter what ailments you have, there are asanas, or poses, that you can do. You can also use yoga accessories, like blocks and straps, to make the poses easier for you. Some of us have sensitive knees and wrists, so it's difficult to put pressure on them, we feel it in our joints. I found an amazing yoga mat, the Maji mat, that solves this problem. It has memory foam strategically placed to make poses much more comfortable. You can find the Maji mat on DharmaSmart.com along with many other useful yoga accessories and yoga gear.

YOGA

A few basic tips:

- Find a flat, open space, where you are free to move around without bumping into anything.

- Set aside at least 30 minutes, and preferably an hour, to devote to this practice and nothing else. Turn off the phones.

- Don't practice on a full stomach. Allow time to digest before exercising. If you are pregnant, or have back problems, consult your doctor before starting any new exercise program.

- Wear loose, comfortable clothing, and bare feet.

- Don't overdo it. Rest when you feel tired. Your stamina will increase over time with regular practice.

- Breathe. Breathe through your nose. Your breaths should be long and deep. Breathe with your diaphragm. Relax your chest and allow your breath to feel as if it is coming from your belly.

- Start out slowly, allow your body to warm up.

- Have fun. Laugh. Enjoy being together. Don't take yourself too seriously.

- Cool down gently, allow your body time to rest and restore itself after you are done.

	VATA	PITTA	KAPHA
FOCUS OF PRACTICE	Calming, grounding	Cooling, relaxing	Energizing, releasing
RECOMMENDED ASANAS (POSES)	Sun Salutation Lotus, Lion, Tree, Triangle, Warrior, Inversions, Cobra, Tortoise, Boat, Twist, Corpse	Moon Salutation, Triangle, Half Moon, Shoulder stand, Boat, Fish, Bow, Tortoise.	Sun Salutation, Lion, Half Moon, Downward Dog, Upward Dog, Handstand, Headstand, Shoulder stand, Plow, Camel

◦⊛ AYURVEDIC MASSAGE (ABYHANGA) ⊛◦

Ayurvedic massage offers many benefits. If done in the morning, it helps you to start your day off relaxed, which is essential in maintaining balance. When done at night, it promotes a restful night's sleep. It doesn't matter when you choose to do the massage, but you will receive the optimum benefits if you do it every day. Since the quality of Vata is dry and cold, a warm and oily massage provides an ideal balance for Vata types, though all types will notice increased health and vitality, especially during Vata season. The massage soothes the nervous system and the endocrine system, since skin produces endocrine hormones. It moisturizes and rejuvenates the skin, promoting a youthful appearance. It also helps the skin to eliminate toxins and tones the muscles.

Sesame oil is generally recommended for Ayurvedic massage because it helps to balance all three of the doshas. But feel free to choose one of the oils that are specific to your dosha. Sesame or almond oil is great for Vata. Coconut or sunflower both work well for Pitta. Corn or olive oils are beneficial for balancing Kapha. You can also add herbs or fragrances to the oils to personalize them for your needs. The entire massage requires only about 2 ounces of oil each time.

Before you begin, warm the oil to skin temperature. The easiest way to do this is to keep a small plastic squeeze bottle filled with oil, and set the bottle in a bowl or cup of very hot water. Wait a few minutes for the oil to reach skin temperature.

While the oil warms, lay out a towel to protect the carpet or floor from any oil that may spill.

When you are ready, start the massage at your head. Drizzle a small amount of oil onto your scalp and massage it in with the palms of your hands. (You can skip the scalp part of the massage on days that you are not washing your hair.) Use a clockwise, circular motion. Then gently massage your face and ears. If you have oily skin, avoid those areas that are prone to breakouts. Massaging the ears is excellent for balancing Vata.

Drizzle some oil in your palms and massage your neck, then move to your shoulders. Use a circular motion on your joints - shoulders, elbows, knees - and long up-and-down strokes on your limbs.

Be gentle on your torso. Use large, clockwise motions to massage the chest and stomach area.

Reach around to massage your back as best you can without straining.

Then massage the legs, ankles, and knees. Using the palm of your hands, vigorously massage the feet.

It is best to leave the oil on the body for 20 minutes before washing it off in a warm, not hot, shower or bath. You can use this time to meditate or do your Yoga exercises. If you don't have time to wait, that's fine. It's much better to do a quick massage than none at all.

WEEK 1
SPACE

DAY 1
∘❦ KITCHEN MAKE-OVER ❦∘

It's been said that the kitchen is the heart of the home. And with good reason! In the past, before we had central heating and air conditioning, the hearth was used both to cook the food and to heat the home. This is where we gather with our families to share meals and to share ourselves. Since we spend so much time here, our kitchens should be warm and welcoming. The kitchen needs to be clean, because this is where we prepare our food. And it needs to be organized so that we can find things easily and we can cook with less effort and more joy.

Today we're doing a kitchen make-over. Don't worry, this is not a complete remodel, just a little freshening-up. It's just a 4-step process, and it's a good idea to go through it at the beginning of every season. So because Ayurveda has 3 seasons, you will want to do this three times a year. This is important because what you see in your kitchen will affect your food choice decisions every time you go in there. Will your kitchen tempt you with junk food, or will it inspire you with fresh, colorful, amazing gifts from nature?

- Starting with the refrigerator and freezer, go through and throw out any food that has expired. Look for the "best if used by" dates on the packages and jars. Go shelf by shelf and make sure you catch everything. Too often we have sauces or crackers that we bought and intended to use, but then forgot about. There's no reason for them to be taking up valuable space when they're old and unusable.

- While you're at it, take a good look at your choices. Read the labels to check for the sugar and fat content. Know what it is that you're eating. If you like to have fortified cereal for breakfast, look for one that is low in sugar and high in fiber. Get rid of any cereals that are high in sugar and low in fiber. Be on the look out for any processed foods, with preservatives and additives. Is this what you want going into your body? If not, toss it, give it away and don't look back.

If you've been drinking soft drinks, one big favor you can do for yourself is to quit now. Do the research and you'll see the toll that all the additives in these drinks take on the body. It doesn't matter if the soda pop is caffeine free, sugar free, diet or whatever, there is no soft drink that is good for you. If you like the fizz, try adding a splash of fruit juice to sparkling water. There are some great machines now, including the "Soda Stream" that will turn your regular water into sparkling water. I have one and I love it! You can make your own sparkling water at home and you'll save money and also help the environment by not having to use all the plastic bottles.

- Now that the shelves are a lot more clear, take everything else out and do a deep clean. Use plain water, or some of the eco-friendly cleaning products that we talked about in Chapter 4. While you're going, take time to enjoy the sparkle, and know that you are creating a little haven for your food.

- Next, it's time to organize and take inventory. Pastas, rice and grains in one area, canned goods in another area, cereals in another area, and crackers and snacks in another area. In the refrigerator keep like items together, and make sure you have plenty of room to store fresh fruits and vegetables.

Also take stock of what containers you have to store food in. When you make your own dips and sauces and dressings you will want to put them in a container where they are easy to see what you have and how much of it you have. Make a list of the kinds of containers, the sizes and number that you need to be efficient in your kitchen.

Take a look at what recipes you would like to try, and what ingredients you have and which you need for those dishes.

- Take your list with you, and go shopping. Items like nuts, rice and beans are less expensive when you buy them in bulk from the bins. Plus, by shopping this way you're saving on unnecessary packaging. Bring your own bags, both the fabric shopping bags and your leftover plastic and paper bags from other purchases to re-use and recycle. Then when you get home, transfer those items from the bags to your containers for neater storage, and save the bags for your next trip to the store. Label your containers with the date you bought each item so you can keep track of what is fresh the next time you go through the cupboards.

DAY 2
◦❊ MEDITATION SPACE ❊◦

You've already set time aside in your schedule for meditation, now it's time to set aside some space for it, too. When we have a regular space to meditate, it's easier for us to get into that settled feeling that allows us to transcend our thoughts. Find a space where you feel comfortable. You can sit on a chair, or sit on the floor on a pillow. Most people like to have some back support, so you can prop a pillow up against a wall, or invest in a specially made meditation chair that is low to the ground and allows you to sit cross-legged if you choose to do that.

Make sure the area where you meditate is clutter free, and that there are no distractions around. You may choose to light a candle, or burn some incense, so it's nice to have a little table nearby. Keep a meditation shawl or scarf in the space, so that it helps up all of the lovely meditative energy, and you can carry this with you when you travel.

Understand that meditation is a practice. Consistency is important, and when you have your own meditation space to go to you are more likely to get into the routine. Make sure it looks beautiful, that it is somewhere you want to go to, and enjoy being.

DAY 3
❧ SLEEPING AND WAKING ☙

Sleep is one of the three pillars of health, so today we are going to create a sleep sanctuary. Follow the guidelines in Chapter 3 to get started.

Consider the setting in which you get yourself to sleep. Is your bedroom more like an office, or an entertainment center? Has your closet spilled out into the room? Are you getting into a freshly made bed or tucking yourself in under messy covers? Are there too many pillows on the bed, or has your pet taken over so that there's no room for you?

Think about how you are waking up. What is the first thing you hear in the morning? Do you wake to a blaring alarm, or the commute report? Wouldn't it be nicer to wake up with light, or with music that you love? There are so many great alarm clocks now, including ones that gradually light up to simulate the light of the rising sun. One reason that Ayurveda recommends that we wake before sunrise is because this is Vata time, and because Vata deals with movement, it helps to get your body going. Once the sun comes up, sometime around 6 am, it's Kapha time, time to get moving and exercise! If you're already up, this is much easier to do.

What is the very first thing you do when you wake up? Rather than just bounce out of bed, think about starting the day with a little poem, or a little prayer of gratitude. You could choose an affirmation for the day, or week, or month and post it on your bathroom mirror to remind yourself every morning.

After you brush your teeth and clean your tongue, splash your face with cool water. This helps to disperse leftover Pitta and prepare the skin for the day ahead. Morning hydration is very important. Rinse your mouth with cool water to get rid of the trapped heat that has dried out the mouth during the night.

DAY 4
⊶ INDOORS/OUTDOORS ⊷

So many times we're stuck indoors. Whether it is because of the weather, or our work schedules, we don't have the opportunity to get out into nature as much as we would like. Today we're going to find ways to bring the outdoors in!

First of all, let in some natural light. Wherever possible, open up curtains and open up windows to let the air circulate. In the winter, when the days are shorter and we don't get enough natural light, you might want to install some full-spectrum light bulbs. These bulbs help to simulate the light of the sun so that we avoid Seasonal Affective Disorder, or SAD, which is a common type of depression that comes from natural light deprivation.

Bring in some greenery. Plants not only make for a more comfortable environment, they also provide much-needed oxygen into your space. Studies have shown that people who work in offices with plants are more productive, and generally happier on the job.

Think about what other things represent nature to you. The sound of water can be very soothing, so you might want to install a little fountain somewhere. Or you can bring in the element of water with a fishbowl.

Seashells, rocks, feathers, and flowers are all items that help to remind us that we are connected to nature. You can start a little collection and keep a bowl on your coffee table or desk. When you need to get grounded, hold one of the items in your hands, and imagine yourself on the beach, or in the mountains, wherever this particular object from nature might have originally come from.

DAY 5
∘⋙ COLOR ⋙∘

Color is an important part of our everyday lives. We use it to decorate our homes and we wear it in our clothing. Color is also a part
of our health. When someone is sad, we say they're "blue." When
they're feeling fine, they're "in the pink." When we feel angry, we
"see red." And optimists are often accused of looking at the world
through "rose-colored glasses." When harnessed, the energy of
color is it is an effective and powerful healing tool.

There are seven colors of the rainbow: red, orange, yellow, green,
blue, indigo, and violet.

In the body, there are seven chakras, or energy centers. Each chakra
corresponds with one of the seven colors. By keeping the chakras
in balance, the body is kept in balance and is healthy.

The first chakra is at the base of the spine. It corresponds with
red. Red is traditionally associated with strength, vigor, sexual
love, danger, and charity.

Near the top of the lumbar area of the back is the second chakra,
which corresponds with orange. Orange is associated with happiness, adaptability, attraction, plenty, and kindness.

The third chakra is located near the solar plexus and corresponds
with yellow. Yellow is associated with mental effort, charm, confidence, persuasion, joy, and comfort.

The fourth chakra is near the heart, and it corresponds with green.
Green is associated with health, wealth, luck, fertility, energy, and
growth.

The fifth chakra is in the throat and corresponds with blue. Blue is
associated with communication, understanding, tranquility, truth,
devotion, sincerity, health, and patience.

In the middle of the forehead is the sixth chakra, which corresponds with indigo. Indigo is associated with ambition, depression,
changeability, impulsiveness, and dignity.

The seventh chakra is at the top of the head, and it corresponds with violet. Violet is associated with spirituality, sentimentality, power, and sadness.

Generally speaking, in color therapy, warm colors (reds and oranges) are used to stimulate. Restaurants and hotels often use these colors in their decor because they are known to stimulate the appetite. Cool colors (blues and greens) are used to calm. Hospitals and doctors' offices frequently use these colors to make people feel more at peace in their surroundings.

In Ayurveda, color is also used to help us to stay in balance. Vatas do best around warm, calming colors like green and yellow. Pittas thrive with cooling colors like blue, white and silver. And Kaphas respond to the stimulating colors of red, orange and gold. With this in mind, I designed beautiful tee-shirts in dosha balancing colors, and you can find them at WearLuck.com.

Today, take a look and see where you can use some color in your home, or in your wardrobe to help you maintain your Perfect Balance.

DAY 6
◦⊶ LESS IS MORE ⊷◦

Our life is frittered away by detail... simplify, simplify.
- Henry David Thoreau, Walden

We could all do with less stress. The more we simplify our lives the less stress we'll have. We don't need so much stuff, first of all. Think of all the time and energy we spend taking care of our stuff. And how much of it do we really use anyway? Think about all the stuff you've got sitting around, in closets, cupboards, drawers – even in plain sight that is basically just collecting dust. That's stagnant energy. Feng Shui likes to have that chi energy able to move around. If our drawers are stuffed to the max and we can't move the hangers around in the closet to see what we have, there's no room to welcome in anything fresh, new, anything that we might really love and want to use.

Isn't it better that all of this stuff, which is likely is pretty good shape and perfectly useful, find a home with someone who really could use it? There are so many great places that accept donations and that will distribute your items to people who really need them.

So today, we purge. You'll be surprised at how much has accumulated over the years. It is so freeing to just let it all go! Bask in the glory of the beautifully arranged stuff that you really do love, and want to keep. You can see it all, and get to it more easily and quickly so you'll actually use it more.

DAY 7
◦∞ HOME AWAY FROM HOME ∞◦

Home is the place where we feel most comfortable, where we can really be ourselves. At home we're surrounded by things that represent who we are, what we like, what makes us feel good. We can create that kind of an environment anywhere that we spend time. Whether you work in an office, in a cubicle, or even out of your car, you can personalize the space to make it more "you."

Is this space clean, organized, clutter-free? Have you included some of the elements of nature there? Does it smell good?

When you travel you can make your hotel room more like home by bringing your meditation shawl with you. You can also bring some aromatherapy essential oils in your favorite fragrances. I always bring almonds and dark chocolate with me when I travel. I never know what food will be available when. Having the comforts of home around helps us to feel more relaxed, and less stressed wherever we go.

Today, pack a little kit that you can take with you in your car, keep in your desk at the office, or throw in a carry-on bag. Think about what items you can carry with you to make any place you go more comfortable.

WEEK 2
BODY

DAY 8
∞ LISTENING TO THE BODY'S SIGNALS ∞

The body is like a tuning fork. It is sensitive to all of the energies in us and around us. It picks up on things way before the brain can process them. Ayurveda tells us to only eat when we're hungry. The body tells us when we're hungry, and we have to pay attention to the signals that it gives us. Today is about listening to the body, reading the signals that it is sending to us, subtle and otherwise.

When we're nervous, often our hands shake, or we get the feeling of butterflies in the stomach. The heart might beat a little faster. We might sweat, or get a dry mouth. When we meet someone we like, we get a warm, relaxed feeling. We find ourselves smiling without even thinking about it. We can use the signals that our body gives us as a kind of barometer when making decisions. When you don't know what to do, which direction to go, tune into the body and see how you feel about each option.

Some call it a "gut instinct" and others call it "following your heart." It's a kind of intuition that shows up physically. Today, throughout the day, check in with your body. Ask it questions and see what kind of a response you get. Try going somewhere, and then close your eyes for a moment, and tune in. What do you feel? What signals is your body giving you? Are any emotions coming up? Pay attention to any answers that come into your head. You're not just making things up, you're learning how to be more in touch with yourself in any given situation. When you can do this you can take better care of yourself.

DAY 9
◦« THE FIVE SENSES »◦

The body is connected to the world through the five senses. These senses help us to stay in present moment awareness. When we're worried or stressed, it tends to be that we are thinking about, or regretting something from the past – or that we are anticipating or concerned about something that might happen in the future. Bringing ourselves into present moment awareness, where we know we are fine right here and now no matter what we are going through, helps us to cope. This moment is the only time there is. We can't live in the past or the future, we can only live in the here and now. Here are some ways you may choose to engage your senses today:

TASTE: To fend off the craving for "sweet" try one little lifesaver type of candy. Really taste it. Close your eyes to make the flavor more intense. Feel it on your tongue. Make it last. Fully experience the taste. You can make this a total meditation really being in the moment as you savor the flavor. When the candy is all gone, know that this is enough. Craving satisfied, completely in a new moment and attention on something new.

SMELL: Experiment with aromatherapy. Breathe in a variety of fragrances, close your eyes, and see how each one makes you feel. Lavender is relaxing, and can help with sleep. Sandalwood is cooling. Rose helps to calm the emotions and works on the heart center to heal emotional pain. Orange is energizing. Try a few and tune in and see how these fragrances affect your body

TOUCH: Get tactile. Stroke your cat, finger-paint, or go barefoot on the grass. Hug someone. The skin is the largest organ on the body and it is so sensitive to texture, and temperature. Get "in touch" with your feelings!

SOUND: Let the music move you! Crank up the tunes and dance around the kitchen. Lose yourself to the rhythm, spin around and get silly. Sit by a fountain and listen to the water. The sounds of nature can be so soothing. Be still and listen. Do you hear the birds singing, the wind blowing?

SIGHT: Take a walk in a lovely garden. Visit a museum, or visit a virtual museum online. Look out the window and reconnect with nature for a little bit. Do a visual meditation.

DAY 10
⟞ HEAD, HEART, HANDS ⟝

It's hard to tell which comes first, the thought, the feeling, or the action. Something moves us, and then we get a thought to do something about it, and then we take action. Or, we have an idea, take it to heart, and then take action. Or, our instincts kick in and we take action almost automatically, before we have a chance to think about it, and then we have to process our feelings about it. The head, the heart, and the hands all work together. The body is our instrument. Today tune into your instincts, see if you can define how you feel, come up with a word for it. Look at the actions you take. Are your head and heart in agreement? If not, which one wins out?

DAY 11
⊸⊛ NATURE'S CALL ⊛⊸

Ayurveda explains that our bodies have certain natural urges that are necessary for our good health. When we suppress these urges we can create health problems. For example, when we feel thirsty, we need to drink. If we don't drink, we can get a headache, fatigue, bladder pain, and more. If we don't eat when we're hungry we can get low blood sugar, light-headedness, and put out our digestive fire. If we don't cry when we feel the need to cry, those suppressed emotions can lead to heart disease. Suppressing our yawns can harm the nervous system. Suppressing a burp can result in hiccups, or even difficulty breathing. So the advice that Ayurveda gives us is to heed nature's call. Let the body function the way it needs to function. Of course, when we do burp, it is proper to excuse ourselves if we are in someone's company!

Today, pay attention to nature's call, and see how it serves you.

DAY 12
⊶ FEELING FATIGUED? ⊷

Who among us doesn't feel stressed out these days? We have plenty of reasons to! Ayurveda says that fatigue comes from on overuse, misuse, or non-use of the mind, emotions, or body. Overuse is overwork, and we do this a lot. Misuse is when we know something is bad for us, but we do it anyway – this can happen with relationships that engage our emotions in a strenuous way. And non-use also causes fatigue because our whole physiology is equipped for "use it or lose it." So if we don't engage our muscles, our minds, and our emotions, they can fade away.

We need to remember that the "stressed out" feeling is not the way we are intended to live. Instead, we are living in our true nature and expressing ourselves fully when we experience a flow of calm energy in the mind and body. So, today we're taking the first step to figure out what you're doing to cause your fatigue, so you can cut it out! Meditation is good for both preventing, and overcoming, any kind of fatigue. Also, eliminate caffeine and work to set your body clock into a natural cycle of rest and activity. Ayurveda has further recommendations for us to deal with fatigue:

- Mental fatigue is caused by an excess of Vata through mental activity, worry, and anxiety. Follow a Vata lifestyle routine to help recover.

- Emotional fatigue is caused by an excess of Pitta through anger, guilt, ambition, and desire. Follow a Pitta lifestyle routine to help get over it.

- Physical fatigue is caused by too much Kapha. Make sure you balance rest and exercise, work and play. Follow a Kapha diet and lifestyle routine.

How are you feeling today? Do you have the energy you require to get everything done that you need to get done? Or are you a bit tired, or run down? What is the cause for this fatigue, and what can you do about it? Take some action steps and see if that helps to bring your energy level up.

DAY 13
◦❀ HEAD MASSAGE ❀◦

According to Ayurveda, massage can help us looking and feeling both youthful and healthy. It gives a beautiful luster to the skin, and tones and relaxes the muscle tissue. Massage improves circulation and thus increases body heat. It also helps the body to release toxins and removes stiffness from the joints, improving nerve supply to the organs and all parts of the body. Massage can improve our concentration, increase our stamina, and make us feel more active and energetic. Ayurveda recommends we do a self-massage (abhyanga) every day. And when we can, it is also beneficial for us to have a head and neck massage, too. Today is the day to indulge the head, give it a little special attention. Here are some tips to get started:

- Pour warm oil on the point that is on a central hair parting, eight finger widths above the eyebrows.

- Massage the oil down both sides of the scalp towards the ears.

- Pour oil on the central crown point, three finger widths behind the crown chakra point.

- Massage the oil onto the scalp towards the ears.

- Tilt the head forward, pour oil onto the back of the skull at the top of the neck.

- Massage the oil along the sides of the scalp towards the back of the ears.

- Use both fists to gently tap the head all over. This stimulates both the circulatory and the nervous system.

- Gently pull some tufts of hair from the roots to relieve muscle tension that keeps the head feeling tight.

- A clockwise motion is recommended for massage as it releases tension.

- Using four fingers, stroke up the back of the neck. Use the right hand for the left side of the neck and the left hand for the right side of the neck.

- Use down strokes on the front of the neck. Do not put pressure on the windpipe.

DAY 14
∘« THE MORNING WALK »∘

You'll notice that in our daily routine I've included a morning walk. This is an important part of the Ayurvedic lifestyle and The Perfect Balance Diet. So as you embark on your walk today, know that there are very valid reasons behind this. Ayurveda recommends a walk in the morning as one of the best ways to start your day, and as a safe and easy way to get some exercise. As we breathe in that fresh, morning air, we take in much-needed oxygen. As we notice the beauty around us, we connect with nature and nourish our creativity. Regular brisk walking can lower cholesterol levels, stimulate circulation, strengthen the heart, and reduce blood pressure. Walking is also a great way to charge up your circulation and boost your metabolism.

In addition, a regular morning walk can fend off stress and depression, help to prevent osteoporosis, and helps us to develop strength, stamina and endurance. Walking doesn't call on blood sugar for energy, and the brain is nourished by blood sugar, so walking is great exercise for the brain. In Ayurveda, morning is known as "brahmmahurat" and is considered the most auspicious time of the day. A little morning sunshine provides us with some Vitamin D. Be sure to drink plenty of water before and during your walk to stay hydrated. And, as always, pay attention to the signals that your body gives you; don't overdo it.

WEEK 3
MIND

DAY 15
◦⊷ BRAIN HEALTH ⊶◦

According to Ayurveda, there are three equally important aspects to mental performance -- "dhi" - learning and comprehension, governed by Vata dosha, "dhriti" - processing and retention of knowledge, the realm of Pitta dosha, and "smriti" - memory or recall, controlled by Kapha dosha.

For the best mental performance and realization of the fullest mental potential, each of these three factors individually needs to be at its peak, and, more important, the coordination among the three factors also needs to be optimal. Ayurveda recommends paying attention to the three fundamental pillars of good health -- food, sleep and relationships -- to achieve this state of mental wholeness and balance.

For today, the challenge is to learn something new. Increase your vocabulary, or learn a phrase in another language, or sign up for a class you've always wanted to take. Whatever it is you choose to learn, engage the brain!

DAY 16
◦❖ PEACE OF MIND ❖◦

Ayurveda explains that our state of mind is instrumental in the condition of our health and well-being. Ayurveda also gives us advice on how to cultivate a healthy state of mind so that we can live a balanced and healthy life. Here are a few suggestions for things you can do today for your peace of mind:

- Take in positive impressions. This can be a challenge in our western culture as we are often inundated by negativity. Seek out uplifting and inspiring works that make you feel good about life in general.

- Release negative emotions. Holding on to negativity can be toxic. Find healthy outlets for emotions so that they don't eat away at you.

- Feel good about yourself and who you are. Develop positive self-worth and self-esteem.

- Keep in mind that the ultimate goal in life is awareness, or moksha.

- Surround yourself with beauty and harmony in your home.

- Take time for rest and time to just be happy.

- Get some sunshine and fresh air daily. Use full spectrum light bulbs in the darker winter months.

- Spend time in nature. Take walks, garden, smell the flowers.

- Visit natural bodies of water, a river, the ocean, a creek or a waterfall.

- Spend time in silence, meditate, chant, or pray.

DAY 17
⌁ A RESPONSE TO STRESS ⌁

As much as we might like to, there's no way we can live a "stress free" life. This is just the world we live in. There is always going to be something stressful happening in the world. It can be huge, like a war, or it can be simply inconvenient, like running late for a meeting. We can't stop stress. But we can change the way we respond to stress. When we respond with fear, our levels of the hormone cortisol rise, and that leads us to experience anxiety, and this affect us both mentally and physically. Stress can literally make us sick.

Fear and anxiety often come with the territory of the busy, complicated lives we lead. They have become a part of our culture. We worry about money, relationships, career, and potential loss. We long for security and guarantees, but in life there are none. So no wonder we are anxious! We are focusing on factors outside of us that are uncertain and unreliable. According to Ayurveda, it is this outward seeking that is the cause of our anxiety. We want control, we want to make things go our way, or to bring about the results we want. Yet even when we get what we want, we are dissatisfied because it doesn't live up to our expectations. We always end up wanting more, and there is no end to it.

What can we do? Surrender. Look within. Remember the truth. Today, focus on what is really important in life, what really matters to you. Approach life without demand or expectation. This may be easier said than done given the bad habits that we've gotten ourselves into! But having anxiety is a big clue that our lives have gotten out of balance, that we are out of harmony with nature. Anxiety shows us how we create discomfort for ourselves. We can use this as a tool to get back on track, back on the path. Meditation helps us to cut through the illusions of the mind.

There are many actions we can take to help lower our cortisol levels, to counter-balance the effects of stress. Besides meditation, we can play with our pets. Cuddling animals helps us to produce oxytocin, endorphins, and other hormones that support self-healing. This is why many hospitals have pets come to visit patients. They're good medicine! Laughter has been shown to lessen pain. Norman Cousins says in his book Anatomy of An Illness that when he was suffering with his illness, he would watch comedies, and "laughter had an anesthetic effect and would give me at least two hours of pain-free sleep."

Creativity is another way we can relax and shake off the effects of stress. We each have ways of expressing ourselves creatively, whether by cooking, writing, painting, knitting, building, gardening or whatever. These activities help to slow us down, help us to become engaged and unaware of the passage of time.

Socializing is also beneficial in helping to us feel better about things. Research shows that people who are lonely have twice the rate of heart disease as people who aren't lonely. Being amongst friends, being part of a group, having functions or gatherings to look forward to – all of this goes a long way towards helping us focus on what makes us feel good, rather than what makes us feel stressed-out.

You may not feel any anxiety, fear, or worry right this second. But it's good to have an action plan for when these emotions come up. In that moment we tend to just react, and typically that reaction is one that has been a habit. So think up an affirmation for yourself that will help you to pause, breathe, and think before you respond. Just like we have learned "Stop, Drop and Roll" when faced with the danger of a fire on us – we can learn "Pause, Breathe, and Think" when faced with those very scary feelings of anxiety.

DAY 18
∘⊷ MENTAL HEALTH ⊶∘

Mental health is an important aspect of Ayurveda. Everything is connected, mind-body-spirit, so one aspect affects all the others. Ayurveda recommends certain techniques to keep mentally fit so that we can function optimally. Today we will remember that we have the freedom to choose our mental states, so we can practice keeping our minds in good shape.

- Meditation. Meditate regularly. Every day, twice a day, for 20-30 minutes each time.

- Cultivate a constructive mental attitude. Develop optimism, cheerfulness, and the habit of possibility-thinking. Remember that challenges are temporary, so don't let them get you down.

- Use your powers of intelligence. Pay attention to your intuition, and look for synchronistic events; there are no coincidences. Choose your words with the best of intention, and speak constructively. Act with purpose to support ordered thinking.

- Keep memories in perspective. There is a difference between the information that we garner from memories and the emotions that are attached to those memories. We can access our memories without having to be influenced by feelings of anger, sadness, guilt, or regret. We can allow memories of success to remind us of the goodness of life. We can let memories motivate us to make better choices in the present moment. Live in the moment, and not in the memories.

- Witness your emotional and mental states rather than becoming identified with them. Remember that these states come and go, so focus on thinking rationally and being emotionally balanced and mature.

- Live with purpose. Have intention behind your actions, and develop constructive habits. Focus on what is important, and what is real. Live the knowledge that you learn. My friend Mallika Chopra started the website Intent.com. Here you can put your intentions in writing and set them free into the Universe! You will find support for your intentions from the other members, and you can support others in their intentions. It's a beautiful community.

DAY 19
◦⊸ WHAT ARE YOU THINKING? ⊷◦

Ayurveda explains our thought process by breaking it down like this:

- Manas is the mind. It senses things outwardly. It relies on the external to give it an impression to focus on.

- Buddhi is intelligence. It perceives both inwardly and outwardly. Buddhi can reason, and put together information based on what we see and what we feel.

- Chitta is consciousness. It feels internally, instinctively, with its own sense of deep knowing.

In addition, there are collective and cosmic counterparts of the mind. The collective is the sensory activity of everyone on Earth. We can sense this, and the media broadcasts some of this. The cosmic is the sensory activity of all creatures in all worlds over all of time. We can connect to the cosmic through meditation.

Today, observe your thoughts. Be the observer, the witness to your thoughts. Think about what you are thinking about – and why. Notice how your thoughts affect you. Direct your thoughts to what you want to pay attention to.

DAY 20
◦«« MANTRA »»◦

"Mantra" is a Sanskrit word meaning "instrument of the mind." It's a tool we can use in meditation to keep distractions at bay. Ayurveda recommends meditation for everyone. And there are specific mantras that are helpful in pacifying each dosha. Today, try using these mantras in your meditation, saying them silently to yourself. Or sing them as you're driving to work, or cooking dinner.

- Ram (pronounced Rahm) is the mantra for Vata. It helps to boost the immune system, and it alleviates fear and anxiety.

- Shrim (pronounced Shreem) is the mantra for Pitta. It promotes general health and harmony.

- Hum (pronounced Hoom) is the mantra for Kapha. It is both stimulating and clearing.

DAY 21
⌀⟐ LEARNING STYLES ⟐⌀

We each have a dominant learning style, the way that we learn the easiest, a style that suits our mind and way of thinking the best. Today look at your learning style, and see how it fits with your dosha, and how you might use this information to help yourself learn, recall, and remember.

Vatas learn quickly, but they then forget quickly as well. It is helpful for Vatas to write things down, and carry a day-planner or a smart-phone app organizer with them all the time. Vatas learn best by listening. A good technique for studying is to listen to a book on tape while reading along. Pittas have a good, sharp, general memory. Pittas are visual learners, so it is helpful for them to have charts, graphs and pictures to refer to. They will remember something better if they read it rather than if they hear it, so keep "to do" lists for them. Kaphas take more time learning things, but once they learn them, they don't forget. Kaphas learn best by association, so tell them stories that relate to the lesson at hand, or give examples of experiences they can remember which apply to what they need to learn.

WEEK 4
SPIRIT

DAY 22
❖ BEHAVIOR RASAYANAS ❖

Rasayana means "recommendation." The following Behavior Rasayanas are for all of the doshas. It is said that following these instructions will help us to avoid contradictions in the mind and therefore prevent physiological strain. They are a reminder of the simple things we can do to help ourselves, and, in turn, to help the world. Today, be mindful of these behaviors, and see how you can, or can better, incorporate them into your life.

- Be honest and kind.

- Be free from anger.

- Abstain from immoderate behavior.

- Be nonviolent and calm.

- Observe cleanliness in yourself and your environment.

- Be charitable toward others.

- Observe a regular daily routine.

- Be loving and compassionate.

- Be respectful, especially to teachers and elders.

- Keep the company of the wise.

- Be modest, have good manners.

- Follow your religious beliefs; be self-disciplined.

- Keep a positive outlook.

- Devote yourself to the development of higher states of consciousness.

DAY 23
∘⋙ SWASTHYA ⋘∘

Swasthya is a Sanskrit word that translated means "established in oneself." This is joyfulness, contentment, and perfect health. In our hectic lives it seems that swasthya is elusive. We look for joy outside of ourselves, in our work, or with our relationships, or even with money. We think that more is better, and put our focus too much on the goals ahead of us, without noticing all the beauty that is among us right where we are. Fortunately, we can change our mindsets. Joy is within us!

One way we can tap into that joy is with meditation. When we quiet our minds, we releases the stresses that have accumulated, and allow the mind and body to get the rest it needs. We can further reap the benefits by supplementing our practice with aromatherapy, herbal teas, warm baths, and massage. It's all a part of taking care of ourselves, of finding that balance that helps us to function optimally. We also need to be mindful of what we put into our bodies. Today, drink lots of fresh water to cleanse and moisturize the entire system. And make an extra effort to eat fresh, nourishing foods. Most importantly, don't postpone happiness. Do what you love to do. Be in a place of gratitude. Spend time with loved ones.

DAY 24
❖ IT'S BLISS! ❖

Ananda means bliss is Sanskrit. Bliss helps to keep us healthy, both mind and body. It feels good! Like laughter, it boosts our immune system and actually heals us. So how do we get more ananda in our lives? Ah! Be loving. That's the simple answer. Today, mindfully practice "ahimsa," or nonviolence in thought, speech and action. Sound easy? Pay attention. Are you thinking gentle thoughts, or does that snarky comment come to mind? What thought could you replace it with? If you think that snarky comment, can you manage not to speak it? What could you say instead? Do you go out of your way to avoid an opportunity to be helpful, or do you go out of your way to move towards it?

Eating fresh, wholesome foods that are easier to digest also helps us to increase ananda. Following an Ayurvedic daily routine helps us to stay stress-free and sleep better. And the best things we can do to increase ananda is to meditate twice a day. Meditation allows us to experience the bliss that is an essential part of who we are. It helps us to have better health, improved relationships, and a calm and clear state of mind. Ananda is a quality of pure consciousness, and it is our natural state of being.

DAY 25
◦⬧ THE COMPASSION BOOM ⬧◦

Karma Yoga is the path of work, activity and service. And now it seems that service is becoming a positive trend! According to the Federal Corporation for National and Community Service, we are experiencing a "compassion boom" right now. It seems that in the past, when economic hard times his, there was a decrease in volunteerism. But today, many more people are participating in public service.

PARADE magazine recently conducted a poll that showed that people feel strongly that service is an essential part of achieving both community and national goals. 90% of those responding said that working hard to teach their children the importance of activism. We are giving of our time and talents in many ways, and even though finances are tight, we're also giving our money. 87% of people polled supported a cause financially in the last year. Interestingly enough, the internet has made it easier to be of service. Many of us are using e-mail, Facebook and Twitter to get the word out about a cause.

When we start shifting our focus to looking within, we understand more and more how we are all connected. And when focus internally, we also see and appreciate how much we have. It is natural for us to want to reach out and give to others, to help relieve some suffering, to bring a little joy to another person. Take some time to give – to give of your time, your talents, and/or your treasure – to give of yourself. That's the best gift of all. And what you'll notice is that you feel like you are the one receiving the gift. It's such a good feeling to give. And not only does it feel good emotionally, giving activates the relaxation response, so it helps to boost the body's natural self-repair mechanisms.

Today, take a look at how you can make a difference, and where you can serve. I'm a Big Sister, with Big Brothers Big Sisters in my community. It's an amazing organization, and I love every aspect of volunteering as a mentor. There are so many great organizations that thrive because of their volunteers. Every single one of us counts, and together we can create the change we want to see.

DAY 26
∘⊰ PURPOSE ⊱∘

When we talk about "purpose" I think that we each have our individual purpose, a reason why we're here in this specific place and time; and that's up to each of us to figure out for ourselves. And then generally, we all have the same purpose, which is three-fold:

- To learn and grow. It seems to be our natural instinct to progress in this way. We can't grow backwards! We look for opportunities to better ourselves, and we find them in our relationships, in classes, in books. We practice behaviors that help us to understand who we are. We look within. Journaling is an example of a way for us to keep track of our thoughts, dreams and desires. It's also a way that we can look back and see how far we've come. Spiritual growth is a strong desire, one that propels us forward.

- To express ourselves and our unique gifts. We are not meant to sit in a shadow and be quiet. We have something to say, both literally and figuratively. So, just what are these unique gifts that we have to share with the world? It's personal for each one of us. To find what this is for you, look at what you love to do. Look at where you love to spend your time. Look at what comes easily to you. There is your talent. Now share it! It takes all of us, and all of our varied and diverse talents, to make this world function.

- To help each other and serve. Many times this goes really well with the second part, and we can use our talent to help others. For example, my mother loves to crochet, and she can whip up a blanket in no time at all. She and a group of her friends at the Senior Center knit and crochet items for children in hospitals. Helping feels good. It's really a gift we give to ourselves. And we have so many chances everyday to really make a difference in the world.

Today think about your unique gifts, and how you can share them with the world.

DAY 27
⋄⊷ THE SOUND OF SILENCE ⊶⋄

From the moment we wake up in the morning, to the clock radio or the alarm, we are inundated with sounds. Phone calls, conversations, newscasts, meetings, traffic, the microwave - it's all there, imposing on our eardrums without us even being aware of it most of the time. What portion of the day do we actually spend in silence? When do we have time to tune in to our own thoughts? Meditation is awesome, and so healthy for us in every way. During the day we can also find little pockets of time to escape the noise of the world. Try this today: when you get in the car, turn the radio off. Just drive without any music or talk shows playing. At first it might be a challenge, we're all kind of "programmed" to have this soundtrack follow us throughout the day. But soon you'll find that it's so much more refreshing to have that little space of peace. Silence really is golden.

And if you think you can do it, try making this a "media fast" day. No computer, no news. Just peace, silence, quiet. Check in with yourself and see how you feel. Are you okay with this, or are you feeling a little restless? A break every once in a while from all the clutter that can come with sound is good for the spirit.

DAY 28
ᴏ◈ GRATITUDE ◈ᴏ

Relationships are one of the three pillars of health in Ayurveda. Make it a point to show affection and gratitude today. With your family members and close friends, this can be a hug. Physical contact (within the boundaries of etiquette) breaks down barriers and brings us closer together. We feel comforted when another human being shows us compassion. People at work can get a handshake or a pat on the back. In ancient times, a handshake was to show an absence of weapons. Now a handshake shows a welcoming, a camaraderie. We all need congratulations. Recognition from our peers on a job well done is a great reward. Offer pats-on-the-backs, literally and figuratively, freely. Smile! And certainly, when someone smiles at you, smile back.

Show appreciation for a person's good qualities. When you get good service in a restaurant, leave a good tip. Be generous. If a coworker has been especially helpful with a project, point that out to the boss. Express gratitude. We don't say "thank you" often enough, or loudly enough! The most appropriate way to show gratitude is to put it in writing. Take the extra time to write a thank you note or to return a favor with a thoughtful gesture. Show affection today for all the good in your life, and gratitude for all the healthy and helpful relationships in your life.

CHAPTER 9

RECIPES FOR AN ENLIGHTENED LIFESTYLE

Nothing will benefit human health and increase
the chances for survival of life on Earth
as much as the evolution to a vegetarian diet.
–Albert Einstein

There are so many reasons why people choose to eat a plant-based diet. First of all, it makes sense, because this is how our bodies are constructed. The act of eating starts with the hands and the mouth. Herbivores have teeth that are more flat, designed for grinding and chewing food. We don't have the sharp canine-type teeth meant for eating flesh that carnivores have. Because meat-eating animals tend to swallow their food whole, they don't need the molars or side-moving jaws that humans and herbivores have. The human hand is suited to harvesting fruits and vegetables. We don't have the sharp claws needed to kill prey.

Our digestive system is another indicator that we as humans are meant to live with a plant-based diet. Once swallowed, meat needs digestive juices high in hydrochloric acid in order to get broken down. Carnivores produce twenty times the hydrochloric acid that herbivores do. The intestinal tracts of herbivores and carnivores also very different. Meat goes back very quickly, so it needs to get out of the body quickly. Carnivores have much shorter digestive tracts than herbivores. When meat goes into the very long (12 times the body length) digestive tract of a human, it takes a much longer period of time to go through the system, which can produce many toxic effects. This puts a strain on our kidneys. When we're young this isn't such an issue, but the older we get the greater risk we face of kidney disease.

The pancreas is also stressed by meat. Animals in nature eat their meat raw – but as humans we cook our meat, which destroys the natural enzymes present in meat that help digestion. This forces the pancreas to produce more digestive enzymes, gradually weakening it.

Of course, there are also all of the physical ailments that are tied to a diet that includes a lot of animal fats. Carnivores can metabolize cholesterol much more easily than herbivores. Over time, when there is a build-up of cholesterol in our systems we get those fatty deposits on the inner walls of the arteries. This plaque constricts blood flow to the heart, which can lead to heart attacks, strokes, blood clots and more. Studies have also shows a correlation between colon cancer and a meat-based diet. In addition, when we eat meat our bodies are forced to process any hormones, antibiotics, tranquilizers and other drugs that these animals have ingested as part of being prepared for slaughter.

The one argument I hear again and again against vegetarianism is that people need their protein. Well, let me assure you that there are plenty of plant-based sources of protein available to us! The elephant, the bull, the rhinoceros and the gorilla are all very content, strong and capable creatures that are also vegetarians. Grains, beans, and nuts are all concentrated sources of protein that contain more protein per ounce than meat.

It is a part of the destiny of the human race,
in its gradual improvement, to leave off eating animals,
as surely as the savage tribes have left off eating each other
when they came into contact with the more civilized.
-Henry David Thoreau

As enlightened citizens, we also need to consider the effects that our food choices make on the planet. John Robbins is the author of Diet for a New America and he is the president of the EarthSave Foundation. He says: "A reduction in beef and other meat consumption is the most potent single act you can take to halt the destruction of our environment and preserve our natural resources. Our choices do matter. What's healthiest for each of us personally is also healthiest for the life support system of our precious, but wounded, planet."

Did you know that 90% of all the grain produced in the USA is used to feed livestock? The USDA's Economic Research Service states that it takes sixteen pounds of grain to produce just one pound of meat. In addition, it takes more than 5,000 gallons of water to produce one pound of beef. And yet it takes just 25 gallons of water to produce a pound of wheat. All of this stresses the earth's resources. On a per acre basis, it just makes more sense economically to grow vegetarian food for people to eat, rather than for to grow food for animals that are bred as food for people. If we instead used these precious resources, the land, grain, and water, to produce vegetarian foods, we would have plenty enough food to feed everyone in the world.

In India, many people, even today, consider cows to be sacred. Although there is much hunger in this country, people would never kill a cow and eat it. One reason for this is that it understood that a living cow gives more food to society than a dead one: milk, cheese, butter, yogurt and more.

From a purely practical standpoint, we can all save a lot of money going vegetarian! Meat is expensive. A family could save hundreds of dollars a year by switching to a plant-based diet. That all adds up to an immense savings over the course of a lifetime. Think of all the extra things you could do with that money.

> *Everyone is God's creature,*
> *although in different bodies or dresses.*
> *–Srila Prabhupada*

One very good reason people often have for going vegetarian is for compassion. Keeping in mind the law of relationship that says, "we are all connected," that means animals as well – all living beings. We share this earth with the animals. We can extend kindness to them, and allow them to live according to their nature the way they were intended to live. I'm sure you've heard all the horror stories about slaughterhouses, and the conditions that animals suffer when they are bred as food. The movie "Fast Food Nation" gives some insight as to what happens at these places, but it's a "cleaned up" version of the harsh reality.

Being vegetarian, or vegan, is just smart all around. Famous, and intelligent, vegetarians include: Pythagoras, Da Vinci, Rousseau, Shelley, Tolstoy, Wagner, Gandhi, George Bernard Shaw, and H.G. Wells. It's also very cool to be a vegetarian! Today many celebrities have embraced a plant-based diet, including: Brad Pitt, Drew Barrymore, Ryan Gosling, Kim Basinger, Dustin Hoffman, Dr. Dre, Paul McCartney, Joaquin Phoenix, Melissa Etheridge, Christy Turlington, and so many more.

Consider trying a plant-based diet. I think you'll see, and feel, the difference and become an advocate of this lifestyle choice just as I am. Even if you can just start with one day a week, hop on the "Meatless Monday" bandwagon and open up your mind, heart, and taste buds to the wonders of creations available to us without harm to our animal friends.

Over the years I've collected and created some amazing recipes. Many of the recipes have been contributed by my friends, family, and subscribers. If you have a recipe that you would like to share with our community, please post on the CoffeyTalk.com website. You'll find many more recipes there, and most are vegetarian or vegan. I like to call these recipes "Flexitarian" because you can use ingredients that you like and are comfortable with using and eating. To me, recipes are just a guideline. Allow yourself to be creative as you cook, improvise like a jazz musician would!

Vegan means no dairy, and no eggs, which can be a challenge in baked goods. But luckily for us, there are many alternatives, and these alternatives are not only good, they are good for us! Soy milk, rice milk, or almond milk is most often used in place of regular milk, and the measurements are the same. To replace eggs, here are some suggestions:

Soy Yogurt. ¼ cup soy yogurt = 1 egg. Use plain yogurt, or for a sweeter taste, vanilla yogurt. This substitution works best in breads, muffins, and cakes.

Extra Firm Silken Tofu. Use a blender to mix the tofu with a splash of soy milk until it is smooth and creamy. ¼ cup blended tofu = 1 egg. This works best with dense cakes and brownies.

Bananas. ½ well mashed banana = 1 egg. Keeps your baked goods nice and moist, but does leave the banana flavor. Works best in breads, muffins, cakes or pancakes.

Egg Replacer. There are some various brands, one is "Ener-G!" 1 ½ Tablespoon egg replacer well mixed with 2 Tablespoons water = 1 egg. This works best in cookies, or items that you want to get crispy.

Flaxseeds. Finely grind the seeds, or have them pre-ground and keep them in the freezer as they are highly perishable. Flaxseeds are a great source of omega-3s. 1 Tablespoon flaxseeds beaten together with 3 tablespoons water = 1 egg. Flaxseeds have a very earthy taste, so they work best in whole grain items like oatmeal cookies.

BREADS, MUFFINS, AND BREAKFAST DISHES

Stewed Apples

This is the perfect Ayurvedic breakfast! Fruit is best eaten first thing in the morning. And fruit is more easily digested when it is cooked. Add in all the wonderful spices, and you've got a tri-doshic treat that fills you up and gets you ready for your big day!

INGREDIENTS:

- 4 tablespoons ghee (clarified butter)
- 7 apples (I like Fuji, but Granny Smith are good, too)
- Sliced almonds, and/or chopped walnuts to taste
- 1/2 cup raisins (I like golden raisins)
- 1/2 cup brown sugar
- 2 teaspoons cinnamon
- 1/4 teaspoon nutmeg
- 1/2 cup water

INSTRUCTIONS:

In a 10" skillet (w/lid) melt ghee over medium heat; turn off heat. Mix in sugar and brown sugar, cinnamon, nutmeg, raisins and the nuts and add ½ cup water, stirring to combine. Bring mixture to a boil and allow to boil until beginning to thicken. Reduce heat to medium; stir in apple slices, turning to coat. Cook over medium to medium high heat 4-5 minutes, stirring, allowing sauce to continue to thicken. Reduce heat to low, cover apples and cook until tender, stirring occasionally, another 5-10 minutes, adding more water if necessary, until apples are tender (cooking time will depend on the thickness of your apple slices). Sauce will thicken as it cools.

Cinnamon Spice Muffins

Cinnamon, spice and everything nice! You can make this vegan or vegetarian – just switch out the milk and eggs with vegan versions. Check out the egg substitutes in the beginning of the chapter and see what you think.

INGREDIENTS:

- ¯1 3/4 cups flour
- ¯1 1/2 teaspoons baking powder
- ¯1/2 teaspoon salt
- ¯1/2 teaspoon allspice
- ¯1/2 teaspoon cinnamon
- ¯3/4 cup milk (I like to use Vanilla Soy Milk)
- ¯1 egg
- ¯1/3 cup oil
- ¯3/4 cup sugar
- ¯1/2 cup butter or margarine, melted (I use Earth Balance vegan butter or ghee)
- ¯3/4 cup brown sugar
- ¯3 teaspoons cinnamon

INSTRUCTIONS:

Heat oven to 350 degrees. Grease muffin pan or line with paper liners. In a medium bowl, combine thoroughly milk, egg, oil, and sugar. Add flour, baking powder, salt, allspice or nutmeg, and cinnamon, and stir to just combine. Fill muffin pan 2/3 full and bake for 20-25 minutes. Combine cinnamon and sugar for topping; set aside. Remove from oven and immediately dip tops in melted butter; then in cinnamon- sugar mixture previously combined. Makes 9-11 muffins.

Breakfast Frittata

This Frittata is really great on a cold morning, hot out of the oven. You can choose other vegetables, any kind you like. You can even switch out the cheese. I've done a version of this same dish with broccoli and cheddar cheese instead of the zucchini and mozzarella.

INGREDIENTS:

- 1 1/2 cups frozen hash brown potatoes
- vegetable oil non-stick spray
- 1 1/2 cups shredded mozzarella cheese, or soy cheese (I use Daiya vegan cheese shreds)
- 1/4 cup nutritional yeast
- 1 cup shredded zucchini
- 2 large fresh tomatoes, chopped (I like Roma tomatoes)
- 1 package firm silken tofu
- 1/4 cup soy or almond milk
- 1 teaspoon basil

INSTRUCTIONS:

In a skillet, cook up the potatoes, and zucchini with a little bit of olive oil. In a bowl, mix the tofu and the shredded cheese together with the nutritional yeast. Add the veggies to the bowl and mix all together. Spray an 8x8 cake pan with veg-oil. Put the mixture in the pan. Bake at 350 for about 40 minutes or until the center is firm. Serves 4-6.

Banana Bread Oatmeal

According to Ayurveda, we're not supposed to mix fruit with dairy. Fruit should be eaten just on its own for the best digestion. But soy products are not considered dairy, so we can do that here! Bananas are a great source of potassium. This is a hearty and delicious breakfast, and the pecans give it an extra punch of protein.

INGREDIENTS:

- 3 cups soy or almond milk
- 3 tablespoons firmly packed brown sugar
- 3/4 teaspoon ground cinnamon
- 1/4 teaspoon salt (optional)
- 1/4 teaspoon ground nutmeg
- 2 cups oats (quick or old fashioned, uncooked) – I like the Irish steel cut oatmeal best.
- 2 medium-size ripe bananas, mashed (about 1 cup)
- 2 to 3 tablespoons coarsely chopped toasted pecans
- Vanilla soy yogurt (optional)
- Banana slices (optional)
- Pecan halves (optional)

INSTRUCTIONS:

In medium saucepan, bring milk, brown sugar, spices and salt to a gentle boil (watch carefully); stir in oats. Return to a boil; reduce heat to medium. Cook 1 minute for quick oats, 5 minutes for old fashioned oats, or until most of liquid is absorbed, stirring occasionally. -Remove oatmeal from heat. Stir in mashed bananas and pecans. Spoon oatmeal into six cereal bowls. Top with yogurt, sliced bananas and pecan halves, if desired.

Vegan Brown Rice Pudding

This recipe is from Cindy Garcia, one of our subscribers. It's an amazing dish, that can really be eaten any time of day. Thanks, Cindy!

INGREDIENTS:

- 1 1/2 cups vanilla almond milk
- 1 Tbsp. cornstarch
- 2 cups cooked brown rice
- 1/4 cup maple syrup (you can use less)
- 1 organic apple, chopped
- 1/3 cup organic whole almonds
- 1/2 teaspoon cinnamon
- 1/4 teaspoon nutmeg
- 1/4 teaspoon ginger
- 1 teaspoon vanilla

INSTRUCTIONS:

Whisk milk and cornstarch together in a medium saucepan. Add cooked rice, maple syrup, apples, almonds, cinnamon, nutmeg, and ginger. Simmer over medium heat for 4 minutes, stirring constantly. Remove from heat and stir in vanilla. Let sit for at least 15 minutes to allow it to set. Chill if desired or serve warm.

Substitutions:

This recipe originally called for 1/3 c. raisins, but I used apples instead. You can probably use blueberries or any fruit you'd like - experiment!

Note It tastes best the next day straight from the fridge!

Nanny's Pancakes

My mother's grandmother made these special German style pancakes for her, and my mother has carried on the tradition in our family. My sons Freddy and Brian can eat about six of these babies each so I have to double or triple the recipe when they come over!

INGREDIENTS:

- 2 eggs
- 1 cup flour
- 1 cup milk (soy or almond milk is okay)
- 2 tablespoons melted butter
- 1/2 teaspoon salt
- Cinnamon
- Sugar

INSTRUCTIONS:

Beat eggs well, beat in milk, salt, flour and butter, cover, let stand 30 minutes. Heat over a skillet or crepe pan until moderately hot, then film with butter using a ladle or small cup, pour in several, then batter, then quickly tilt pan so it spreads evenly. When batter looks dry, flip to get the other side fully cooked. Sprinkle with cinnamon and sugar and roll up. Top with more cinnamon and sugar.

Breakfast Pizza

This recipe was contributed by Kate Simone, a CoffeyTalk subscriber. She uses real cream cheese and sausage, but I've "veganized" the recipe! Super easy, and also a great after-school snack.

INGREDIENTS:

- 1 lb. meatless "sausage" – there are many varieties to choose from, including Boca.
- 1 8 oz. container soy cream cheese, softened
- 1 can of refrigerated crescent rolls
- Vegetables you enjoy
  (Kate likes: 1 onion, 1 red pepper and 1 yellow pepper)

INSTRUCTIONS:

Brown the sausage and drain. Cook any vegetables on which you and the kids can agree. Mix together sausage, veggies, and softened cream cheese. Unroll the crescent rolls and spread flat on a cookie sheet or pizza tin. Spread cream cheese mixture on top. Bake according to directions on the package of crescent rolls.

Crunchy Granola

Whenever I make this recipe I can't help but start singing the Neil Diamond song "Crunchy Granola Suite." Definitely takes me back! I don't know if granola was actually invented in the '70's but I remember eating a lot of it growing up. This is my take on it – and it's great to make up a bunch and have it on hand to use in other recipes, too! My favorite combo is sliced almonds, dried blueberries and sunflower seeds.

INGREDIENTS:

- 3 Cups Rolled oats
- 1/4 cup Wheat germ
- 1/8 cup Honey
- 1/8 cup Vegetable oil VARIATIONS: ADD YOUR FAVORITE COMBINATIONS
- 1/2 cup raisins OR ½ cup dried apricots, cranberries, blueberries or other dried fruit
- 1/4 cup slivered almonds, OR ¼ cup cashews, peanuts, or walnuts
- 1/8 cup unsweetened shredded coconut
- 1/8 cup sesame or sunflower seeds

INSTRUCTIONS:

Preheat oven to 300F. Grease a large baking sheet with edges. In a large bowl mix oats together with wheat germ. In small saucepan heat honey and oil until honey is thin and runny. Add mixture to oats and blend well. Spread granola thinly and evenly on baking sheets and bake about 15 min, or until lightly browned. Cool. Spoon into a large bowl, add raisins or the rest of your ingredients, and mix thoroughly. Store in a tightly covered container and keep in a cool dry place.

Black Bean and Sweet Potato Hash

Our subscriber Chrissie contributed this recipe online. Really flavorful and nutritious!

INGREDIENTS:

- 1-2 T. olive oil
- 2 c. chopped onion
- 2 garlic cloves, minced
- 6 cups peeled diced sweet potatoes (1/2 pieces)
- 1 jalapeno, minced
- 1 T. ground coriander
- 1 T ground cumin
- 1 t. salt
- 1 c. frozen corn (or 1 can)
- 1 ½ c. cooked black beans (15 oz. can)
- splash of water or orange juice
- cayenne or hot pepper sauce (opt.)

INSTRUCTIONS:

Heat oil in large, deep, skillet or pot. Add the onions and sauté on medium heat, stirring occasionally, until they begin to soften. Stir in the garlic, cook for a few seconds, then add the sweet potatoes. Add the jalapeno, coriander, cumin, and salt. Add the corn and black beans and a splash of orange juice (opt). Mix. Cover and bake in a 350 oven 45-60 minutes until sweet potatoes are softened. (Or simmer on the top of the stove until done). Add cayenne or hot pepper sauce if desired. (Optional: you may serve this with chopped cilantro or minced scallions and a dollop of sour cream or yogurt.)

Vegan Cornbread

My friend Missy Hughes is a southern belle who has now made her home in California. She's been able to bring the flavors of the south together with the healthy vegan lifestyle with this amazing cornbread recipe!

INGREDIENTS:

- 2 tablespoons ground flax seed
- 6 tablespoons water
- 1 cup all-purpose flour
- 1 cup cornmeal
- 1/4 cup sugar
- 4 teaspoons baking powder
- 3/4 teaspoon table salt
- 1 cup soy milk
- 1/4 cup canola oil

INSTRUCTIONS:

1. Adjust oven rack to middle position; heat oven to 425 degrees. Spray 8-inch-square baking dish with nonstick cooking spray. 2. Bring the water to a boil in a small saucepan. Add the ground flax seed, reduce the heat to medium-low, and simmer the ground flax seed in the water for 3 minutes or until thickened, stirring occasionally. Set aside. 3. In a medium bowl, whisk together the flour, cornmeal, sugar, baking powder, and salt until well-combined. 4. Add the ground flax seed mixture, soy milk, and canola oil to the flour mixture. Beat just until smooth (do not overbeat.) 5. Turn into prepared baking pan. Bake for 20 to 25 minutes, or until a toothpick inserted in the middle comes out clean. 6. Cool on wire rack 10 minutes; invert cornbread onto wire rack, then turn right side up and continue to cool until warm, about 10 minutes longer. Cut into pieces and serve.

Blueberry Muffins

This is a recipe I turn to again and again. It's wonderful when fresh blueberries are in season! At other times of the year, try it with dried cranberries and orange zest. Chopped walnuts are optional.

INGREDIENTS:

- 2 cups of flour
- 1 cup of sugar
- 1/4 teaspoon of salt
- 3 teaspoons of baking powder
- 2 large eggs, or equivalent of egg substitute
- 1 cup of soy milk
- 2 teaspoons vanilla
- 1/2 Cup (or one stick) of unsalted (sweet) butter, softened

INSTRUCTIONS:

Preheat oven to 350 degrees Fahrenheit   Mix together dry ingredients. When thoroughly combined, add in 1 cup of fresh blueberries! In a separate bowl, mix together the rest of the ingredients. Make a well in the center of the dry ingredients, pour in the wet ingredients, and mix together just until moist, don't over mix! Scoop into muffin cups lined with paper, or greased muffin tins.   Bake for approx. 40 minutes, or until golden brown. Makes about a dozen extra-large muffins.

Super Moist Spiced Banana Bread

I used to think I made a great banana bread, until I tasted my neighbor Sue Levine's banana bread! My son Brian is best friends with Sue's son Aaron, and he used to go next door and have Sue's banana bread all the time. When Brian went off to college he asked me to send him some, so Sue gave me the recipe. And now I'm hooked! According to Sue, everything tastes a bit better when it's baked with chocolate chips, and I have to agree.

INGREDIENTS:

- 1 1/2 cup sugar
- 2 eggs
- 2 medium ripe bananas, mashed
- 1/2 cup oil
- 1 3/4 cups flour
- 1 teaspoon baking soda
- 1/2 teaspoon baking powder
- 1 1/2 teaspoon pumpkin pie spice
- 1 teaspoon cinnamon

INSTRUCTIONS:

Beat together sugar, eggs, and bananas until blended. Beat in oil, and remaining ingredients until blended. do not over beat (stir by hand) Pour batter into 4 3x5" greased foil loaf pans and bake in a 350 degrees F oven for 40-50 minutes or until a cake tester comes out clean. cool for 10 minutes. remove breads from pans and continue cooling on a rack.

Orange Walnut Bread

I don't know where I found the recipe, but I get so many compliments on this delicious Orange Walnut Bread! It's really nice to bring to breakfast meetings, to keep those growling stomachs at bay.

INGREDIENTS:

- 1 1/2 cups flour
- 1/2 cup sugar
- 2 tsp. Baking Powder
- 1/2 tsp. baking soda
- 1/2 tsp. salt
- 2 eggs, beaten
- 1/4 cup (1/2 stick) margarine or butter, melted
- 1/2 cup orange juice
- 2 Tbsp. grated orange peel
- 2 Tbsp. water
- 1 cup Walnuts, chopped

INSTRUCTIONS:

Mix flour, sugar, baking powder, baking soda and salt in large bowl; set aside. -Blend eggs, margarine, orange juice, orange peel and water in small bowl. Stir into flour mixture just until blended. Stir in walnuts. Spoon into greased and floured 8x5-inch loaf pan. -Bake at 350°F for 50 minutes or until done. Cool in pan 10 minutes. Remove from pan; cool completely on wire rack. Slice; serve immediately.

SOUPS, SALADS, SIDE DISHES AND STUFF

Pear Walnut Salad

I had a similar salad at a fancy restaurant and loved it so much I went home and re-created it! Instead of the Romaine, you could use Arugula if you'd like. Really simple, and when you serve it at a dinner party, very impressive!

INGREDIENTS:

- 1 head romaine lettuce, chopped
- 2 large pears, cut into bite-sized pieces
- 1/2 cup candied walnuts
- 3 stalks of green onions, chopped

Dressing:
- 1/2 cup sesame oil
- 4 tablespoons apple cider vinegar

INSTRUCTIONS:

This salad looks best when arranged on a plate with one thing on top of the other and the dressing drizzled on top. If you're serving a large crowd, just mix it all up in one big bowl instead.

Sunday Salad

I call this salad "Sunday Salad" because my husband loves it so much he wants to have it every Sunday. And it's simple enough that he can make it himself, so Sunday is his day to cook.

INGREDIENTS:

Dressing:
- 1/4 cup rice vinegar
- 1/4 sesame oil
- 2-3 Tablespoons Mellow white miso

Salad Ingredients (the following items are suggestions, choose what you like - be creative!)
- Romaine lettuce, chopped
- Arugula
- Scallions
- Tomato
- Avocado
- Garbanzo beans, or kidney beans
- Peas
- Corn
- Sliced almonds
- Pepitas (pumpkin seeds)
- Chopped walnuts
- Sesame seeds

INSTRUCTIONS:

Put all the salad ingredients in a large bowl. Mix up the salad dressing with a fork until creamy. Toss the salad, and serve with warm crusty bread.

Pomegranate Salad

Pomegranates are hailed as a kind of wonder fruit – and this is something Ayurveda has been aware of for centuries. The Sanskrit name for the pomegranate is "Dadima." The main taste is considered to be astringent, but it also may contain the taste of sweet, sour, and bitter. While the pomegranate is excellent for improving digestion, the beauty is that it doesn't increase Pitta. Best of all, the pomegranate is an aphrodisiac! Ayurveda says that it is a remedy for impotence – eat one pomegranate every night for fourteen nights and you're good to go! They're also great for helping to overcome nausea. Pomegranate seeds are these little jewels just packed with flavor and nutrition – and in this salad, they're the star of the show!

INGREDIENTS:

- 1 cup garbanzo beans
- All the seeds from 1 fresh pomegranate
- 2 cups watercress leaves (heat in a skillet to wilt)
- 1 Tablespoon pine nuts, toasted

INSTRUCTIONS:

Toss all of the above with a dressing of lemon juice and olive oil and a little sea salt. Yummy!

FSA Sprinkles

My friend Michele Santangelo got me hooked on FSA. This mixture has a slightly sweet and nutty taste and can be sprinkled on rice, pasta, fruit, veggies, or just about anything. It is a good source of protein, essential fatty acids, minerals, and fiber and is definitely an anti-aging mixture.

INGREDIENTS:

- 3 cups flaxseeds (also called linseeds)
- 2 cups sunflower seeds
- 1 cup almonds

INSTRUCTIONS:

Mix and grind together until fine. A regular coffee grinder will do the job. Store in a dark airtight glass jar in the refrigerator.

Cranberry and Quinoa Salad

My friend Susan Alburtus contributed this recipe. I originally met Susan through Facebook, and now we compete against each other in Words With Friends all the time. This salad of hers is so colorful and fun – a real crowd-pleaser!

INGREDIENTS:

- 1 1/2 cups water
- 1 cup uncooked, rinsed quinoa
- 1/4 cup chopped red bell pepper
- 1/4 cup chopped yellow bell pepper
- 1 finely chopped small red onion
- 1 1/2 teaspoons curry powder
- 1/4 cup chopped fresh cilantro
- 1 lime, juice d
- 1/4 cup toasted sliced almonds
- 1/2 cup minced carrots
- 1/2 cup dried cranberries
- salt and ground black pepper to taste

INSTRUCTIONS:

Prepare quinoa according to package directions. Cool and put into a bowl and refrigerate until cold. Remove from refrigerator and stir in the other ingredients. Chill well before serving.

Bruschetta

This is a wonderful summertime appetizer, when fresh tomatoes are at their most abundant. I live in California, where we can get fresh tomatoes all year round. Every Christmas I make a big batch of it, the red and green together are very festive! As an option, you can serve the Bruschetta warm, just by throwing everything into a skillet for a few minutes. This is an appetizer my family loves!

INGREDIENTS:

- 8 large, ripe, plum (roma) tomatoes, chopped
- 16 large basil leaves, fresh, finely shredded
- 1 tablespoon chopped garlic
- 1/2 cup extra-virgin olive oil

INSTRUCTIONS:

Combine all of the above ingredients, and serve with toasted rounds of baguette bread. Drizzle with balsamic vinegar or top with toasted pine nuts if desired.

Barley Vegetable Soup

This recipe was contributed to our website by Terry Takahashi. Terry says that she often adds any vegetables she happens to have on hand, and she also swaps out the barley for pasta on occasion. This is a really hearty soup, and super easy to make.

INGREDIENTS:

- 3/4 cup pearl barley
- 11 cups vegetable stock (This is about 2 of the boxes you can find in any store.)
- 2 tablespoons extra-virgin olive oil
- 1 1/2 cups chopped onion
- 1 cup chopped carrots
- 1/2 cup chopped celery
- 1 cup thinly sliced mushrooms
- Salt to taste
- 1/2 bunch parsley

INSTRUCTIONS:

In a saucepan, combine the barley and 3 cups of vegetable stock. Bring to a boil over medium heat, cover, and simmer for 1 hour, or until the liquid is absorbed. Meanwhile, heat the olive oil in a large pot and add the onion, carrots, celery, and mushrooms. Cover and cook the vegetables for about 5 minutes, until they begin to soften.

Note: If you like a soup with lots of veggies, add 1/4 - 1/2 cup of an in season vegetable.

Add the remaining vegetable stock and simmer 30 minutes, covered. Add the barley and simmer 5 minutes more. Add salt to taste and ladle into bowls. Serve garnished with fresh parsley.

Mung Bean Dahl

In Ayurveda, Dahl is a staple. It's one of those perfect foods that fills you up and carries you through the day. Shalimar is one of my favorite restaurants, and they make the best Mung Bean Dahl I've ever had. Every time we go there I get two extra orders to take home with me! Dahl is like a cross between a chili and a soup. If you haven't tried dahl, please do!

INGREDIENTS:

- 1/2 cup split hulled mung beans
- 3-4 cups water
- 1-3 teaspoons ghee (clarified butter)
- 1/2 teaspoon cumin seeds
- 1/8 teaspoon turmeric

INSTRUCTIONS:

Sort and wash the mung beans. Drain.

In a heavy-bottomed pot, add the beans, turmeric and 3 cups water. Bring to a boil; then turn heat down to medium/low and simmer-cook until dhal is butter-soft (about 30-40 minutes). Stir occasionally to prevent sticking, and add more water as needed to maintain desired consistency. If foam forms on the surface, skim it off and discard. When cooked, add salt and stir. In a separate pan, heat ghee until melted to a clear oil. Add the cumin seeds and stir to release aroma. The cumin should turn a rich dark brown but not burn. Pour the ghee-spice mixture carefully over the dhal. Stir and serve immediately with boiled Basmati rice or other whole grain and vegetables.

Fresh Corn and Zucchini Salad

This is a summertime favorite! I love to grill corn outside on the BBQ right next to my veggie burgers. And when my mom plants zucchini, we get an abundance of them!

INGREDIENTS:

- 6 ears corn, cooked, kernels removed from cob
- 2 small zucchini, thinly sliced
- 4 green onions, thinly sliced
- 1/2 red bell pepper, thinly sliced
- 1/4 cup flat-leaf parsley, finely chopped

INSTRUCTIONS:

In a salad bowl, mix together all of the vegetables. Top with your favorite vinaigrette, or make your own fresh dressing with 1/2 cup olive oil and 1/4 cup fresh lime juice.

Artichoke Orzo

This is a great salad to make when you need to take a dish over to someone's house for a potluck. It's especially good when the weather is warm. You can keep it in the fridge and have it as a side dish with just about any meal.

INGREDIENTS:

- 1 cup orzo (cooked according to package directions)
- 1 Tablespoon lemon zest
- 1 Tablespoon lemon juice
- 1 tsp. oregano
- 1 small jar quartered marinated artichoke hearts
- 1/4 cup chopped black olives
- 3 green onions, sliced

INSTRUCTIONS:

Mix all of the ingredients, including the artichoke marinade. Refrigerate until ready to serve, or pack in a plastic container for your picnic!

Lazy Mashed Potatoes

I always thought making mashed potatoes was such a chore because I didn't like peeling potatoes. Then I discovered that if I use the gold, white, or red skinned potatoes, instead of the Russet Potatoes, I didn't have to peel them! Now making mashed potatoes is a snap, and I do it all the time. This is one of Greg's favorite dishes; he loves it when we have leftovers.

INGREDIENTS:

- 3 large Potatoes, white, yellow or red skinned, cut into half, leave the skin on.
- 2 Tablespoon Earth Balance vegan butter
- 1/4 cup chopped green onions
- 1 lemon

INSTRUCTIONS:

Juice the lemon and set aside the juice and the rind. Put the potatoes in a saucepan and cover with salted water. Add the lemon rind and bring to a boil. Reduce heat and cook 30 minutes or until potatoes are tender. Drain off the water and remove the lemon rind. Using a potato masher, mash potatoes and Earth Balance. You can make them smooth, but I like to leave them a little chunky. Add 1 teaspoon of lemon juice, the green onions, and salt and pepper to taste. Stir all together.

Cranberry Chutney

Chutney is a traditional Indian side dish that is almost like a jam. There are many different varieties of chutney. This is one of my favorites. It's especially good during the holiday season, it makes a lovely hostess gift!

INGREDIENTS:

- 1 pound fresh cranberries
- 1 cup water
- 2 cinnamon sticks
- 1/2 teaspoon ground allspice
- 1/8 teaspoon ground cloves
- 1/2 teaspoon salt
- 1 cup dried apricots, chopped
- 1 1/2 cups white sugar
- 1 cup seedless grapes
- 1 cup chopped celery
- 1 large apple, chopped (unpeeled)
- 1/2 cocktail onions
- 4 lemon slices, chopped
- 1/2 cup raw sunflower seeds

INSTRUCTIONS:

Place first group of ingredients in a large saucepan. Bring to a boil, lower heat, and cook until the cranberries burst open. Add the second group of ingredients and bring to a boil. Stir, cover, and simmer for 30 minutes. Remove cover, and cook for an additional 15 minutes until mixture thickens. When chutney is thick, remove the cinnamon sticks, and add the sunflower seeds. Let cool. Keep refrigerated. Serves 6-8

Candied Nuts

I learned how to make these yummy candied nuts when I was in Girl Scouts! One year I made them for everyone for Christmas presents. I put them in little glass jars, and made Santa hats for the jars out of red and white felt. Everyone loved it! You can use any kind of nuts you like. And you can add cinnamon to the mix if you want, too.

INGREDIENTS:

- 1 1/2 cups blanched whole nuts
- 1/2 cup sugar
- 2 Tablespoons butter or margarine

INSTRUCTIONS:

In a heavy skillet, mix the nuts, sugar and butter. Cook over medium heat, stirring constantly, for 6-8 minutes or until the sugar is melted and the nuts are toasted. Spread the nuts onto a buttered baking sheet or a piece of aluminum foil. Separate into bite-sized clusters. Cool.

ENTREES

STIR-FRY MENU

With this super simple stir-fry system you can have a completely different meal every night of the week. Make your own sauce and you avoid all the preservatives and additives that you often find in sauce that you buy already made on the grocery store shelves.

- Make the sauce and set aside.
- Heat about 2 Tablespoons of oil for every 4 servings in a wok or large skillet.
- Brown the protein. Take out of the skillet and set aside.
- Chop up the vegetables and greens into bite size pieces.
- Put the vegetables into the skillet and cook until they are soft, but still bright in color.
- Add in the leafy greens just until they wilt.
- Then add the protein back into the mix.
- Add the sauce to the mixture until everything is well coated and heated.
- Put the carb on the plate, and then top with the stir-fry. Serve.

Oil (Choose 1)	Coconut, Sesame, Olive, Almond, Ghee, Safflower, Sunflower
Carb (choose 1)	Jasmine rice, Basmati rice, Rice noodles, Udon noodles, Quinoa, Millet
Protein (choose 1 or 2)	Tofu (extra firm, cubed), Seitan, Edamame, Almonds, Cashews, Seeds: sunflower or sesame, Gardein "Chicken" – any variety
Vegetables (choose 2 or more)	Asparagus, Bell peppers – any color, Broccoli, Cauliflower, Carrot, Green bean, Peas - any variety, Zucchini, Yellow Squash, Bean sprouts
Leafy Greens (choose 1)	Bok choy, Baby bok choy, Kale, Spinach, Chard
Sauce (choose 1)	Teriyaki sauce, Almond sauce, Tahini sauce, Lemon sauce, Garlic sauce

Teriyaki Sauce

INGREDIENTS:

- 1/4 cup soy sauce
- 1/2 cup water
- 1/2 cup pineapple juice
- 1/2 teaspoon fresh ginger
- 1 clove chopped garlic
- 4 tablespoons packed brown sugar
- + 2 tablespoons cornstarch
- 1/4 cup cold water

INSTRUCTIONS:

Blend the 2 Tablespoons of cornstarch and ¼ cup of cold water and set aside.

In a sauce pan, heat the rest of the ingredients. When heated, add the cornstarch and water mixture. Stir well. If sauce is too thick, add more water or juice until it is the consistency you like.

As an option, you may substitute orange juice, apple juice, rice wine or additional water for the pineapple juice.

Almond Sauce

My husband had this amazing peanut sauce on his stir-fry dish at a restaurant, and I asked our waiter for the recipe and he gave it to me! I'm allergic to peanuts, and peanuts are not generally recommended in Ayurveda, so I adapted the recipe, and also made it easier to make at home. However, note that this recipe makes a LOT of sauce! Just use what you need, and pour the rest into jars to freeze and have on hand for the next time you want to use almond sauce.

INGREDIENTS:
- 1 jar almond butter
- 1 cup rice vinegar
- 3/4 cup Braggs (or lite soy sauce)
- 1 can (approx. 2 cups) CoCo Lopez
- 2 cans (14 oz. ea.) coconut milk
- 1/2 cup dark brown sugar
- 1 1/2 teaspoon ground cumin
- 1 1/2 teaspoon ground coriander
- 1/4 cup garlic puree
- 3 cups almond, or sesame oil

INSTRUCTIONS:
Combine all ingredients in a large bowl and whisk together well. If the almond butter is very thick and hard to blend, heat it up to melt it a little bit first.

Tahini Sauce

INGREDIENTS:
- 1/2 cup tahini
- 1/2 cup orange juice
- 1/2 cup rice vinegar
- 1/4 cup Bragg's

INSTRUCTIONS:

Mix well. When heated this sauce binds together and gets creamy.

Lemon Sauce

INGREDIENTS:
- 1/4 cup fresh lemon juice
- zest from 1 lemon
- 1/4 cup vegetable broth
- 1 Tablespoon Bragg's
- 1 Tablespoon Agave

INSTRUCTIONS:
Mix well.

Garlic Sauce

INGREDIENTS:

- 2/3 cup Bragg's
- 1/2 cup vegetable broth
- 1/3 cup rice wine
- 3 1/2 tablespoons sugar or 2 Tablespoons agave
- 1 tablespoon sesame oil
- 1 tablespoon minced garlic
- 1 tablespoon minced ginger
- 2 tablespoons cornstarch dissolved in
- 1/4 cup water

INSTRUCTIONS:

Put the sesame oil, garlic and ginger in a saucepan and cook 15-30 seconds. Add in the Bragg's, vegetable broth, rice wine and sugar. Bring to a boil, then reduce heat. Add in the cornstarch mixture and return to a boil until the sauce is thick.

PASTA MENU

Pasta is a staple at our home, we have it at least once a week. With so many delicious variations it's a different meal every time. The Italian flag is red, white and green, and I have sauces in each color! You can also make a "pink" sauce by mixing the red and the white sauce. I often add a scoop of the green sauce into the red sauce for a little variety. And you can add the white sauce to the green sauce as well to make a creamy pesto.

Cook up some fresh vegetables, either by steaming, sautéing or grilling, and add to any of the sauces to make a Primavera version. Start with any of these pastas, or pasta substitutes and cook according to the package directions:

Pasta: any shape, in regular, wheat, or spinach

Gluten free rice pasta

Gluten free corn pasta

Spaghetti squash, cooked and scraped out to look like pasta

Soba noodles

Shirataki noodles (made from tofu, packed in water, no cooking required)

Then top with one of these sauces:

Red Sauce

For this recipe you could use 2 large cans of tomato sauce to start, but I prefer using fresh tomatoes. Especially in the summer, when tomatoes are abundant, there's nothing like a fresh tomato marinara sauce.

INGREDIENTS:

- 10-12 Roma tomatoes, blanched and peeled
- 1 small onion, chopped
- 4 Tablespoons olive oil
- 6 cloves of garlic, chopped
- 1/4-1/2 cup fresh basil, julienned
- 1 teaspoon salt
- 1 teaspoon sugar
- 1/2 cup red wine

INSTRUCTIONS:

Put the tomatoes in the blender or food processor until you have them liquefied. In a large sauce pan, sauté the onion and garlic in the oil.

Add in the rest of the ingredients, including the tomatoes, and bring to a boil. Reduce heat and simmer 30-45 minutes until the sauce reduces and thickens up.

White Sauce

This sauce is like an alfredo sauce, but with a lot less fat – and no dairy! You can use it as a creamy base for many other sauces. Just add some tarragon and you've got a Bernaise sauce to use over vegetables or meat substitutes.

INGREDIENTS:

- 1/2 cup raw cashews
- Water
- 1 teaspoon fresh lemon juice
- 2-3 cloves of garlic, chopped
- 1 Tablespoon olive oil
- 2 Tablespoons nutritional yeast

INSTRUCTIONS:

Pour enough hot water over the cashews to cover, and allow to sit overnight. Drain off the water. Pour new water over the cashews to cover, and then put the water and cashews in a blender or food processor. (I use the VitaMix blender – it's a professional quality and so easy to use to mix up anything.) Blend until smooth. Add in the fresh lemon juice, chopped garlic, olive oil and nutritional yeast and blend again.

Green Sauce

This green sauce is a take on the traditional pesto sauce. You can adapt and vary it to your taste. The leafy greens "cook" when they are tossed with the hot pasta.

INGREDIENTS:

- Equal parts:
- Fresh Basil and
- Spinach and/or Arugula
- Olive oil
- Pine Nuts (raw) and/or
- Sunflower seeds (raw)
- Chopped garlic
- Daiya shredded mozzarella, and/or rice or soy grated Parmesan.

INSTRUCTIONS:

Leafy greens shrink up in volume once you put them in the blender, so they're hard to measure. I just go by handfuls. Put a handful of fresh basil, and a handful of spinach and/or arugula in the blender. Add a handful of raw pine nuts and or sunflower seeds combined. Add about 1 Tablespoon of chopped garlic, more or less to taste. I like lots! Next add about ½ cup of your favorite non-dairy cheese. Pour in about ½ cup olive oil and blend. If needed, add more olive oil until sauce is emulsified.

Hawaiian "Chik'n"

INGREDIENTS:

- 1 packages Gardein Scallopini Vegan Chicken Cutlets (4 in a bag)
- 1/4 cup Earth Balance vegan butter
- 1/2 cup orange juice
- 1 T lemon juice
- 1/4 c brown sugar
- 1 1/2 teaspoon arrowroot (you can also use corn starch)
- 1 1/2 t soy sauce
- 1 small can pineapple cubes
- Parsley flakes for garnish

INSTRUCTIONS:

Take Gardein Scallopini Cutlets and dust with flour. Melt Earth Balance vegan butter large skillet. Brown Gardein Scallopini Cutlets for about 2 minutes on each side, remove from pan. Combine orange juice, lemon juice, brown sugar, cornstarch and soy sauce in the skillet. Bring sauce to a boil and continue stirring. When sauce is thickened, add pineapple cubes and the Gardein. Sautee until Gardein cutlets are coated well and heated through. Serve over rice.

Lissa's Famous Vegan Quiche

Anytime I serve this up people say the same thing: "Is this really vegan?" They can't believe it! So creamy and yummy you'll never miss the eggs and cheese. Great as a brunch dish, too.

INGREDIENTS:

- 1 prepared pie crust (I like Marie Callender's brand, it's frozen, you don't have to thaw it out.)
- 1 box Mori Nu Firm Silken Tofu (I use the Lite version)
- 1 bag fresh baby spinach, steamed
- 1/2 - 1 Cup frozen peas, cooked
- 1 bag shredded soy or Daiya cheese, any flavor you like
- 1/2 cup Nutritional Yeast
- Optional: sautéed garlic, onions, your favorite spices.

INSTRUCTIONS:

Preheat oven to 375 degrees. After you cook the spinach, place it on a chopping board and chop it up. In a large bowl, place the Mori Nu Tofu, and break it up with a fork. Add the spinach, peas, cheese, nutritional yeast, and any additional flavorings. Mix all together and pour into the frozen pie crust shell. Bake on a baking sheet at 375 degrees for 50 minutes or until knife comes out clean when poked in the center of the quiche. Let stand about 10 minutes before serving. Enjoy!

Potato Frittata

This frittata is kind of like a quiche, and it's versatile enough to serve for any meal. All you need is a green salad and some fresh bread to go with it and you're done!

INGREDIENTS:

- 1 pound firm tofu crumbled
- 1/4 cup soy milk
- 1/4 cup chopped fresh parsley leaves
- 1/8 teaspoon turmeric
- 1/2 cup shredded soy or Daiya mozzarella
- 1 tablespoon olive oil
- 2 garlic cloves, minced
- 2 large potatoes, baked or roasted and cut into 1/2 inch dice
  OR use a bag of cubed potatoes.

INSTRUCTIONS:

Preheat oven to 400 degrees F. Mix up half the tofu in a food processor (you can also use a blender or a hand beater) along with the soy milk, parsley, turmeric and 1/4 cup of the soy cheese. Process until smooth and set aside. Heat the oil in a large skillet over medium heat. Add the garlic and potatoes and cook, turning occasionally until potatoes are lightly browned on all sides, about 5 minutes. Add the remaining crumbled tofu and the pureed mixture stirring well to combine. Cook until the mixture is beginning to set (3-4 minutes). Transfer the frittata to a baking pan and top with the rest of the cheese. Bake until firm and hot, about 25 minutes. Let stand for about 5 minutes before cutting and serving.

Vegetable Bake

This is made with all vegetables, but you could easily add cubed tofu, seitan, or white beans. Improvise! It's a wonderful main course when served with a hunk of sourdough bread or corn bread.

INGREDIENTS:

- 2 russet potatoes, cubed
- 1 ruby red potato, or yellow yam, cubed
- 1 yellow onion, diced
- 1/2 cup broccoli, chopped into bite size pieces
- 1/2 cup green beans, chopped into bite size pieces
- 1 large zucchini, cut into rounds
- 1 large carrot, cut into rounds
- 1 yellow squash, cut into rounds
- 1/2 cup olive oil
- Dried herbs (basil, oregano, thyme, garlic)

INSTRUCTIONS:

Put all of the vegetables in a roasting pan, toss with olive oil and your favorite dried herbs. Bake at 350 degrees for 45 minutes. Feel free to use whatever vegetables are in season, or whatever vegetables you have on hand.

Pineapple Fried Rice

If you want to get really fancy, you can use fresh pineapple – cut the pineapple in half vertically, leaving the top leaves in place. Scoop out the pineapple, and then use the hollowed out halves as your dishes to serve the Fried Rice in. Makes a beautiful presentation! I'm not a big pepper fan, so I usually omit the red peppers and add raisins. As an option, you can use curry sauce instead of teriyaki sauce, too. Lots of possibilities!

INGREDIENTS:

- 1/4 cup teriyaki sauce
- 8 oz. firm tofu, cubed
- 1 Tbsp. Vegetable Oil
- 1 medium red pepper, cut into strips (about 1-1/2 cups)
- 1/2 cup (1-inch) green onion pieces
- 2 cups Rice, cooked, chilled
- 1 can (8 oz.) pineapple tidbits in juice, drained
- 1/2 cup cashews, chopped

INSTRUCTIONS:

Pour teriyaki sauce over tofu in shallow dish. Refrigerate 5 to 10 minutes to marinate. Drain tofu; reserve teriyaki sauce. Heat oil in large skillet on medium-high heat. Add tofu; cook 3 to 4 minutes or until golden brown on all sides, stirring occasionally. Remove from skillet. Add red pepper to skillet; cook and stir 2 minutes. Add green onion; cook and stir 1 minute. Add rice and pineapple; mix lightly. Cook 2 to 3 minutes or until heated through, stirring frequently. Add tofu, cashews and reserved teriyaki sauce; mix lightly. Cook until heated through, stirring occasionally.

Baingan Bharta

My subscriber Jenifer contributed this recipe. I absolutely love eggplant so this is a favorite. I use soy yogurt, and I omit the chile peppers, but you can make this as spicy as you like. Serve over rice, or with a slice of Naan, Indian bread.

INGREDIENTS:

- 1 large eggplant
- 2 tablespoons vegetable oil
- 1 teaspoon cumin seeds
- 1 medium onion, thinly sliced
- 1 tablespoon ginger garlic paste
- 1 tablespoon curry powder
- 1 tomato, diced
- 1/2 cup plain yogurt
- 1 fresh jalapeno chile pepper, finely chopped (optional)
- 1 teaspoon salt
- 1/4 bunch cilantro, finely chopped

INSTRUCTIONS:

Preheat oven to 450 degrees F. Place eggplant on a medium baking sheet. Bake 20 to 30 minutes in the preheated oven, until tender. Remove from heat, cool, peel, and chop. Heat oil in a medium saucepan over medium heat. Mix in cumin seeds and onion. Cook and stir until onion is tender. Mix ginger garlic paste, curry powder, and tomato into the saucepan, and cook about 1 minute. Stir in yogurt. Mix in eggplant and jalapeno pepper, and season with salt. Cover, and cook 10 minutes over high heat. Remove cover, reduce heat to low, and continue cooking about 5 minutes. Garnish with cilantro to serve.

Vegan Lasagna

When we have our annual board retreat for Big Brothers Big Sisters, this is the dish I bring, and it's one of the first to disappear – everyone loves it! It's one of those meals that look like you worked for hours in the kitchen – but in reality you can whip it up in just a few minutes!

INGREDIENTS:

- 1 package no-boil lasagna noodles (Trader Joe's makes a good one - also Barillla and Ronzoni)
- 1 box Mori Nu firm Silken Tofu
- 3 tablespoons nutritional yeast
- 2 teaspoons garlic powder
- 2 bags veggie shreds Mozzarella "cheese" (or Daiya cheese for strict vegans)
- 2 jars pasta sauce (I like to get mine at the Italian deli - it's made fresh there)
- Optional: 1 bag of fresh baby spinach, cooked
- Pine nuts
- Truffle oil

INSTRUCTIONS:

Spray a casserole dish with non-stick spray. Using a fork, mash up the tofu with the nutritional yeast and garlic powder. This makes the "ricotta" layer.

Layer:

- Sauce / Noodles / Cheese / Noodles / Sauce / Ricotta / Sauce
   Noodles / Cheese / Noodles / Sauce / Cheese

Top with pine nuts and a drizzle of white truffle oil. Let sit on the counter 20-30 minutes so the noodles get a little soft from the sauce.

Bake at 375 degrees F for 45 minutes. Top should be bubbly and hot.

Let sit for 10 minutes to set up before serving.

Chickpea Curry

My husband adores this dish. He mixes up leftovers with salad for his lunch the next day. Chickpeas, also called garbanzo beans, are a great source of protein. Serve this over rice, with a salad or green vegetable on the side. I usually make fresh spinach to go with it.

INGREDIENTS:

- 2 Tablespoons vegetable oil
- 2 onions, minced
- 2 cloves garlic, chopped
- 2 teaspoons ginger root, chopped
- 6 whole cloves
- 1 teaspoon cinnamon
- 1 teaspoon ground cumin
- 1 teaspoon ground coriander
- 1 teaspoon ground turmeric
- 2 (15 ounce) cans garbanzo beans (chickpeas)
- 1 cup fresh cilantro, chopped
- salt and pepper to taste.
- If you like it spicy, use cayenne pepper.

INSTRUCTIONS:

Heat oil in a large frying pan over medium heat – sauté onions until tender. Stir in garlic, ginger, cloves, cinnamon, cumin, coriander, salt, pepper and turmeric. Cook for 1 minute, stirring constantly. -Mix in the garbanzo beans and their liquid. Continue to cook and stir until all ingredients are well blended. Remove from heat. Stir in cilantro just before serving.

Vegan Pot Pie

Hearty, hot, homey – pot pie is everything you want on a cold winter's day! This is a one-dish meal, and so delicious.

INGREDIENTS:

- 1 pack Gardein "Chicken" Scallopini cut into 1/4 cubes (they come frozen, and you can cut them up frozen)
- 1 cup onion, diced
- 1 cup diced potato or sweet potato
- 1 cup frozen peas (frozen is fine)
- 3/4 tsp. thyme
- 3/4 tsp. sage
- 3/4 tsp. sea salt
- 1 tbsp. nutritional yeast flakes
- 1 tbsp. Bragg's liquid aminos
- 3 tbsp. olive oil

Roux:
- 1/2 cup flour
- 1/2 cup Earth Balance Butter
- 4 cups vegetable broth or vegan chicken broth

- Puff Pastry sheets, or tube of biscuit dough, separated.

INSTRUCTIONS:

Pre-heat oven to 375 degrees

Brown Gardein Scallopini in a sauté pan with 1 tablespoon of olive oil.

Season with salt and pepper. Remove from pan and set aside. In a large stock pot, cook onions in olive oil for 3 minutes and add potato, sage, thyme, salt and pepper. Continue to cook for 5 minutes. Put the Gardein chicken and peas into the pot. In a separate pan, make the roux: melt the stick of butter, and then add 1/2 cup of flour. When well combined add the broth until well mixed and boiling. Then whisk in the yeast flakes and Bragg's. Add the roux a bit at a time and continue to cook as sauce begins to thicken. Stir in Gardein Scallopini, Bragg's liquid aminos and peas. Pour mixture into a baking dish. Top the pan with the puff pastry sheets, or pop open the tube of dough and pull the biscuits apart to fit over the top of the dish. Bake for 35-40 minutes, until hot and bubbly and pastry sheets are golden brown.

DESSERTS AND TREATS

Pumpkin Cookies

These cookies signal the start of Fall, when there's a chill in the air and we start thinking about Halloween and Thanksgiving. This recipe makes a lot of cookies, so I share with my Little Sister from Big Brothers Big Sisters. Between our two households they don't last long!

INGREDIENTS:

- 1/2 cup butter or margarine
- 1 1/2 cups sugar
- 1 egg
- 1 cup cooked pumpkin
- 1 tsp. vanilla
- 2 1/2 cups flour
- 1 tsp. baking powder
- 1 tsp. soda
- 1/2 tsp. salt
- 1 tsp. nutmeg
- 1 tsp. cinnamon or 2 tsp. pumpkin pie spice
- 1/2 cup diced almonds, roasted
- 1 cup chocolate chips

INSTRUCTIONS:

Cream together butter and sugar until light and fluffy. Beat in egg, pumpkin and vanilla. Mix flour, baking powder, soda, salt and spices. Add to creamed mixture and mix well. Add almonds and chocolate chips; with heavy spoon, mix thoroughly. Drop by teaspoonfuls onto a well-greased cookie sheet. Bake at 350 degrees for 15 minutes or until lightly browned. Remove from cookie sheet while still warm and cool on rack. Makes about 6 dozen cookies

Granola Cookies

You can use your own home-made granola for this recipe, or I often go to Whole Foods and scoop out a big bag of it to have on hand. A nice cookie/granola bar hybrid.

INGREDIENTS:

- 2 eggs
- 3/4 cup brown sugar
- 3/4 cup white sugar
- 1 cup butter or margarine
- 1 teaspoon vanilla
- 2 cups flour
- 1 teaspoon baking soda

INSTRUCTIONS:

Beat together eggs, sugars, butter and vanilla. Then add in the dry ingredients and blend well. Fold in 2 cups of your favorite granola (I like the kind with dried blueberries in it!) Drop by teaspoonfuls onto an ungreased cookie sheet. Bake at 375 degrees for 10 minutes or until golden brown.

Prize Peach Cobbler

My Grandma Penny left me so many great recipes, but this one is my all time favorite! I've made it so many different ways, with pears, blueberries, apples, even adding in chocolate chips. Use your imagination, and whatever fruit is in season. My sister Marci has perfected the art of the cobbler and brings a different version to every family gathering.

INGREDIENTS:

- 3/4 cup flour
- Less than 1/8 teaspoon salt
- 2 teaspoons baking powder
- 1 cup sugar
- 3/4 cup milk
- 1/2 cup butter or margarine
- 2 cup fresh sliced peaches 1 cup sugar on peaches (optional)

INSTRUCTIONS:

Sift flour, salt, and baking powder, mix with 1 cup sugar; slowly mix in milk to make batter. Melt butter in 8x8x2 pan. Pour over melted butter. Do not stir. Mix peaches and 1 cup sugar cover thoroughly. Carefully spoon them over batter. Bake 1 hour at 350 degrees F. serve hot or cold with cream if desired. 6 servings

Zucchini Cake

I got this recipe from Freddy and Brian's great grandmother, Harriet Henderson. This is one of my favorite cakes, super moist and delicious. It's a sneaky way to get kids to eat their vegetables!

INGREDIENTS:
- 3 eggs
- 2 cups of sugar
- 1 cup vegetable oil
- 3 tsp. vanilla
- 1 lb. grated zucchini (unpeeled) or a bit more.
- 2 cups flour
- 2 tsp. baking soda
- 1 tsp. salt
- 1 tsp. Cinnamon
- 3/4 cup raisins
- 3/4 cup walnuts
- Cream Cheese Frosting:
- 1 container Tofutti Better than Cream Cheese
- 1/2 cup soy margarine
- 2 cups powdered sugar
- 1 tsp. vanilla extract
- 1 1/2 tsp. lemon juice

INSTRUCTIONS:

Preheat oven to 325 degrees F.

Zucchini Cake: Combine eggs, sugar, oil and vanilla and beat them together until the mixture is smooth. Add grated zucchini and stir. Sift in dry ingredients together and add the nuts. Add the dry ingredients to batter and pour into a 9x13 greased and floured pan. Bake for one hour until done. Let it cool before adding the cream cheese frosting.

Cream Cheese Frosting:

Combine the cream cheese and margarine. Slowly add the powdered sugar, then the vanilla and lemon juice. Blend well. Once Zucchini cake is cooled add to the top of the cake.

Vegan Lemon Poppy Seed Cookies

My Little Sister Allysa found this recipe online and now we make these cookies together all the time. They're really quick and easy to mix up. It's so fun to bake together!

INGREDIENTS:

- 3/4 cup sugar
- 3/4 cup brown sugar
- 3/4 cup margarine (butter or ghee)
- 3/4 cup soy yogurt
- 1 1/2 tsp. vanilla
- 3/4 teaspoon baking soda
- 3/4 teaspoon salt
- 1 teaspoon lemon zest
- 2 1/2 cup flour
- 1/3 cup poppy seed

INSTRUCTIONS:

Preheat oven 350 degrees F, mix all ingredients, bake 8-9 minutes until done.

Vegan Cappuccino Cupcakes

I'm a cupcake fanatic! To me there's nothing more festive. These cupcakes are my favorite.

INGREDIENTS:

- 1/3 cup canola oil
- 3/4 cup sugar
- 1/2 cup soft silken tofu, blended until creamy with a little bit of soy milk
- 2/3 cup vanilla soy milk or rice milk
- 4 Tablespoons instant decaf coffee
- 1 1/4 cups unbleached all-purpose flour
- 1 Tablespoon unsweetened cocoa powder
- 1 teaspoon baking powder
- 1/4 teaspoon baking soda
- 1/2 teaspoon ground cinnamon
- 1/2 teaspoon salt
- For Ganache frosting:
- 3 Tablespoons vanilla soy milk
- 1/3 cup semisweet chocolate chips

INSTRUCTIONS:

Preheat oven to 350 degrees F.

Line muffin pan with paper liners. In a large bowl, whisk together oil, sugar, tofu, soy milk, vanilla, and coffee until smooth. In another bowl, sift together the flour, cocoa, baking powder, baking soda, cinnamon and salt. Mix the wet ingredients into the dry ingredients until combined and smooth. Fill the liners 3/4 full. Bake 20-22 minutes. Don't overbake. Cool completely, and frost!

Chocolate Ganache Frosting:

Heat the soy milk in a microwave safe bowl (I use a Pyrex measuring cup) until almost boiling. Add the chocolate chips and stir until they are melted in and blended with the milk. Cool for a few minutes, and then drizzle onto the cupcakes.

Apricot Bars

Diana was like an aunt to me growing up. She introduced me to tacos, hot fudge sundaes, and making noise on New Year's Eve. She's an amazing cook! She taught me how to make these yummy Apricot Bars when I was young, and I'm still making them today! You can use any kind of jam; I like apricot the best, especially when it's my mother's homemade apricot jam.

INGREDIENTS:

- 1 1/2 cup flour
- 1 cup brown sugar
- 1 teaspoon baking powder
- 3/4 cup butter
- 1 1/2 cup rolled oats
- 1 cup apricot jam

INSTRUCTIONS:

Mix everything except jam together until crumbly, put 2/3's of mixture in 11x8 pan   spread with jam. Cover with remaining of crumbs. Bake 375 degrees F for 30 minutes. Cook and cut into bars.

Sticky Toffee Pudding Cake

My husband is Australian, and he introduced me to this fabulous traditional Australian dessert. It's one of those things that you can't just buy in the store; you've got to make it up yourself. And it's so worth it! This is what I usually make for his birthday every year; he loves it.

INGREDIENTS:

- 1 3/4 cups dates, pitted and chopped
- 1 teaspoon baking soda
- approx. 1 1/2 cups boiling water
- 1/4 Cup + 1 Tablespoon cup butter
- 3/4 cup white sugar
- 2 eggs
- 1 1/8 cup self-rising flour
- Caramel Sauce Topping: 1/3 cup butter, or vegan equivalent
- 3/4 cup packed brown sugar
- 2/3 cup evaporated milk
- 1 teaspoon vanilla extract

- If you are vegan, substitute 1/2 cup of plain soy yogurt for the eggs, and use margarine instead of butter.

INSTRUCTIONS:

Preheat oven to 350 degrees F (175 degrees C). In a small bowl, combine the dates and baking soda. Pour boiling water over the dates just to cover them. Cream 1/4 cup plus 1 tablespoon of the butter with the white flour until light. Beat in the eggs and mix well. Add the flour, and the date mixture (including the water) to the egg mixture and fold to combine. Pour the batter into an 8 inch round baking pan. Bake at 350 degrees F 30-40 minutes. Let cool. Slice and serve with warm caramel sauce. To make the caramel sauce: In a small saucepan combine the brown sugar, evaporated milk, and vanilla. Cook over medium heat and bring to a boil. Turn down heat and simmer 5 minutes, stirring occasionally.

AFTERWORD

Full circle. It's a term we hear a lot. Whenever we go anywhere, or do anything, we make progress. This is the nature of life. We step outside of ourselves so that we can experience, explore, discover – and then we bring those experiences back to self so that we learn and grow. And then when we step outside of ourselves again, we bring that newfound knowledge with us, so that we experience, explore and discover more deeply, more profoundly.

In our modern day, contemporary lives we are both blessed and burdened with what might be called "conveniences." Our technology is such that it is not a necessity for us to grow all of our own food as our ancestors once did. We can shop for it anytime. We can even order online and have it delivered right to our door. We can buy it frozen, or canned, because our foods come this way, so that they last longer on the shelves. When we need an answer to a question, we can search the Internet, and not bother going to the library. We can keep up with our friends by their posts on Facebook, so there's no need to "bother" anyone with a phone call. Science has developed techniques and topical treatments to keep us looking ever-youthful – for a price. The modern becomes more modern, updated and upgraded at a rapid pace.

And yet, as time goes on, life does not seem to be getting easier for us; it seems to be getting more complicated. In general, as a society, we're stressed out, overworked, overweight, overwhelmed, and just plain tired. But it doesn't have to be this way. And hopefully now that you've read the book and implemented some of the practices into your life you can see this, too.

Now is the perfect time to continue with using the ancient wisdom that has brought so much beauty and clarity to life. There's no need to forgo any of the progress that helps us to be effective and efficient. We can live an enlightened lifestyle using ancient wisdom with modern style. It's about making choices that clearly define our priorities. We've seen what works, what doesn't work – what makes sense and what doesn't. We can pick and choose and design for ourselves the kind of life that we want to live, that we are meant to live. There's no "perfect" and there's no standard we have to live up to. We know and understand that it is our unique imperfections that make us the perfect individuals that we are. We can find, and live, our Perfect Balance. When we find ourselves on the spiritual path, we learn to become aware of what we think, what we say and what we do. We see how every action we take has repercussions, and meaning. So we naturally strive to be more mindful in every area of life. We are paying attention to where we shop, what we buy, what we wear and how we wear it, and what we eat and how we cook it. Now instead of being merely a consumer, we are taking on the role of being a citizen, and looking at the "big picture." We think about where we go, and how we get there. We take notice of who we meet, and why. Somewhere along the line we discover that our bliss is in our hands, and in our hearts, and we carry it with us at all times.

This book is about coming full circle, getting back to some of the beautiful and practical rituals and traditions that serve us so well. My intent with The Perfect Balance Diet is to show you how you can embrace some of the tried and true wisdom from ancient times and integrate it into your life to bring you more joy, more bliss, every day. It's about understanding our place on this planet, and with each other. Whether we want to be healthier, happier, or more at peace – there are centuries-old principles and practices that we can apply right now, right here where we are.

Enlightenment is lightening-up. Bring in the light and let it shine in you, through you, as you!

ABOUT THE AUTHOR

Lissa Coffey is a lifestyle and relationship expert who serves up an inspiring blend of ancient wisdom and modern style on her website CoffeyTalk.com. She's been living an Ayurvedic lifestyle since researching her first book, "The Healthy Family Handbook," in 1996. Lissa appears frequently on television and radio and contributes to many national publications with her insightful and compassionate approach to modern-day issues. Her e-mail newsletters are enjoyed around the world by a steadily growing subscriber base. She has e-courses through DailyOm.com and Udemy.com.

Lissa Coffey is a certified instructor with The Chopra Center. Deepak Chopra says: "Coffey brings the timeless wisdom of Ayurveda to a contemporary audience and shows us how to discover more about ourselves and our relationships." In 2005 she was awarded a commendation from Los Angeles Mayor Antonio Villaraigosa for her "Outstanding Contribution to the Yoga Community." In 2012 AAPNA (Association of Ayurvedic Professionals North America) awarded Lissa the "Dharma Award" for "Excellence in Promoting Awareness of Ayurveda."

OTHER TITLES BY LISSA COFFEY

What's Your Dharma: Discover the Vedic Way to Your Life's Purpose

CLOSURE and the Law of Relationship: Endings as New Beginnings

What's Your Dosha, Baby? Discover the Vedic Way for Compatibility in Life and Love

Getting There With Grace: Simple Exercises for Experiencing Joy

Getting There! 9 Ways to Help Your Kids Learn What Matters Most in Life

The Healthy Family Handbook: Natural Remedies for Parents and Children (co-authored with Louise Taylor)

Freddy Bear's Wakeful Winter

Feng Shui For Everyday: Easy Ways to Bring Abundance Into Your Home and Workplace

ACKNOWLEDGEMENTS

We're all connected, and we're here to help each other learn and grow. This is the Law of Relationship, and I see it in action every single day. My heart is filled with gratitude to all the teachers I have learned from over the years, especially Louise Taylor, Deepak Chopra, and Vasant Lad.

Much love and gratitude goes to both my family and to my global family. We're all in this together, and your support and encouragement mean the world to me. You inspire me! My CoffeyTalk team gets a standing ovation from me: Ophelia, Brian, and Jon, Chris, Brody, Eric and Ray, thanks for your help every step of the way.

Thank you Bill Gladstone for believing in me and in my work. Thank you Barbara Deal for your faith in me. I am so blessed to have you both in my corner.

And my wonderful husband, my partner, my heart: Thank you for learning and growing with me, for loving me, and for being my cohort on this amazing adventure called life.

REFERENCES AND RECOMMENDED READING

Ashley-Farrand, Thomas, "Healing Mantras: Using Sound Affirmations for Personal Power, Creativity, and Healing" Ballantine-Wellspring, New York, NY, 1999

Chopra, M.D., Deepak, and Simon, M.D., David, and Backer, Leanne, "The Chopra Center Cookbook: Nourishing Body and Soul" John Wiley & Sons, Hoboken, New Jersey, 2002

Chopra, M.D., Deepak, "Perfect Health: The Complete Mind/Body Guide" Harmony Books, New York, NY, 1991

Hospodar, Miriam Kasin, "Heaven's Banquet: Vegetarian Cooking for Lifelong Health the Ayurveda Way" Dutton, New York, NY, 1999

Johari, Harish, "Ayurvedic Massage: Traditional Indian Techniques for Balancing Body and Mind" Healing Arts Press, Rochester, Vermont, 1996

Lad, Vasant, ""Textbook of Ayurveda: Fundamental Principles" The Ayurvedic Press, 2002

Khalsa, Karta Purkh Singh and Tierra, Michael, "The Way of Ayurvedic Herbs" Lotus Press, Twin Lakes, WI, 2008
Khalsa, M.D., Dharma Singh, and Stauth, Cameron, "Meditation as Medicine: Activate the Power of Your Natural Healing Force" Pocket Books, New York, NY, 2001

Iyengar, B.K.S., "Light on Pranayama: The Yogic Art of Breathing" Crossroad Publishing Company, New York, NY, 2002

Levacy, William R., "Beneath a Vedic Sky: A Beginner's Guide to the Astrology of Ancient India" Hay House, Carlsbad, California, 1999

Mastro, Robin and Michael, "Altars of Power and Grace: Create the

Life You Desire"
Balanced Books, Seattle, WA, 2003

Maria, Sarah, "Love Your Body, Love Your Life"
Adams Media, 2009

Pert, Candace, "Molecules of Emotion: The Science Behind Mind-Body Medicine"
Simon & Schuster, 1999

Pert, Candace, "Psychosomatic Wellness: Guided Meditations, Affirmations and Music to Heal Your Bodymind" (Audiobook)
Sounds True, 2008

Prabhupada, Srila, "The Higher Taste: A Guide to Gourmet Vegetarian Cooking and a Karma –Free Diet"
The Bhaktivedanta Book Trust, Los Angeles, CA, 2006

Robertson, Laurel, and Flinders, Carol, and Godfrey, Bronwen, "Laurel's Kitchen: A Handbook for Vegetarian Cookery and Nutrition"
Nilgiri Press, Berkeley, CA 1976

Schäfer, Lothar, "Infinite Potential: What Quantum Physics Reveals About How We Should Live"
Deepak Chopra, 2013

RESOURCES

The Perfect Balance Club
www.PerfectBalanceDiet.com
Menus, recipes, videos, meditations and more!

DharmaSmart: Purposeful Living Essentials
www.DharmaSmart.com
Ayurvedic remedies, oils, herbs and more!

Share Recipes
www.CoffeyTalk.com

What's Your Dosha? Quiz and more
www.WhatsYourDosha.com

What's Your Dharma? Your Life Purpose
www.WhatsYourDharma.com

All About Meditation
www.PSMeditation.com

Dosha Design: Vastu & Feng Shui
www.DoshaDesign.com

Sleep Tips
www.BetterSleep.org

The Ayurvedic Institute
www.ayurveda.com

The Chopra Center
www.chopra.com

Maharishi University of Management
www.mum.edu

SOCIAL MEDIA

YouTube.com/coffeytalk

Facebook.com/perfectbalancediet

Facebook.com/lissacoffeytalk

Twitter.com/coffeytalk

Instagram.com/lissacoffey

Pinterest.com/lissa_coffey

HuffingtonPost.com/lissa-coffey